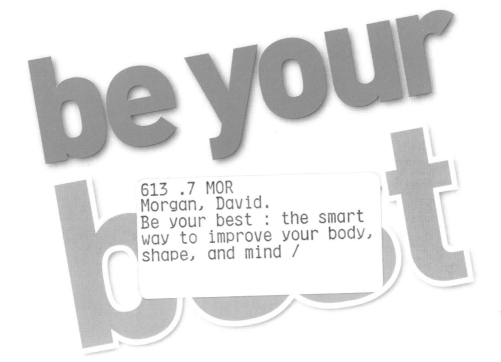

be your best

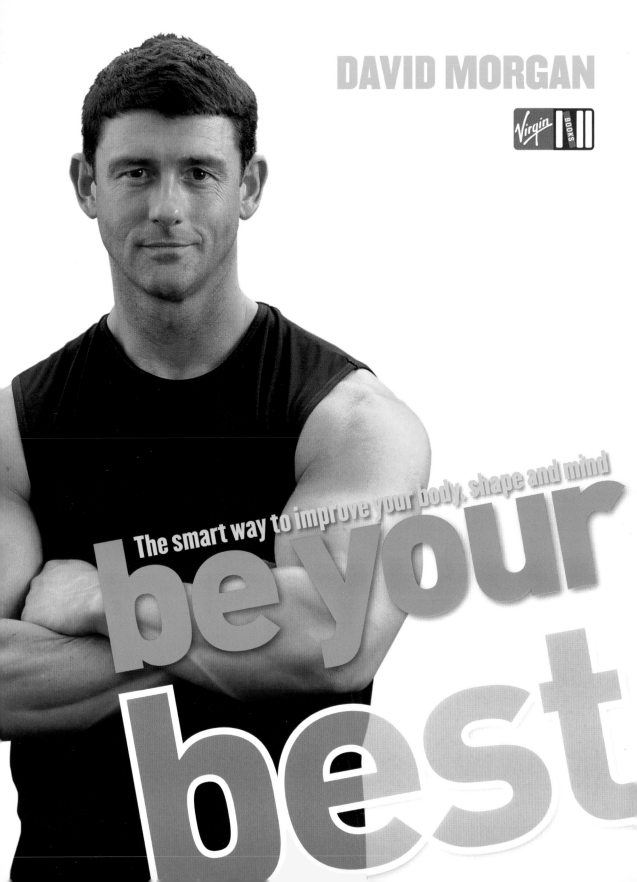

DAVID MORGAN

Virgin BOOKS

The smart way to improve your body, shape and mind

be your best

acknowledgements

Special thanks to Real Public Relations (Cambridge), Paul Flower and his patient wife Onny (remember, it's the long-term benefits), KT Forster (what would have happened if we'd not met at Heathrow?) – and to Sarah-Jane.

visit www.beyourbest-davidmorgan.com

First published in Great Britain in 2007 by
Virgin Books Ltd
Thames Wharf Studios
Rainville Road
London
W6 9HA

Copyright © David Morgan 2007

The right of David Morgan to be identified as the Author of this Work has been asserted by him in accordance with the Copyright, Designs and Patents Act, 1988.

A catalogue record for this book is available from the British Library.

ISBN 978 07535 1199 2 (UK)
ISBN 978 07535 1226 5 (USA)

The paper used in this book is a natural, recyclable product made from wood grown in sustainable forests. The manufacturing process conforms to the regulations of the country of origin.

Designed by Virgin Books Ltd

Photography copyright © Perry Hastings
Illustrations copyright © Andy Roberts

Printed and bound in Great Britain by The Bath Press

contents

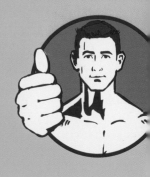

beyourbest

foreword

By Randall J. Strossen, Ph.D. President of IronMind Enterprises, Inc., California.

If you're going to write a successful fitness book, a ready smile and a sharp set of abs can be essential assets, so it's a good thing that David Morgan has both of these.

Going the next step, though, Dave has two qualities that nobody in the world can match: his pattern of success as an Olympic-level weightlifter, and his relentless search for information on how to train more effectively.

In the Olympics, the sport of weightlifting involves two lifts you might never have seen in the flesh – the snatch, and the clean and jerk. Both lifts require tremendous athleticism as well as great strength. If I told you that Dave Morgan cleaned and jerked 205kg as an 82.5kg weightlifter, that might not mean too much to you. But if I said that means while weighing about 181 pounds, he could lift over 450 pounds from the ground to arms' length overhead, you would and should be very impressed.

More remarkable, though, was the fact that Dave Morgan achieved world class status while training with his brother in the family garage at the end of the garden in Cambridge, England. In a sport dominated by the products of the old Soviet sports

machine, Brits, very simply, are not expected to lift the way Dave Morgan lifted. So you can rest assured that Dave Morgan isn't another hollow pedagogue; he was head of the class and his lifting at the Olympics, World Championships and Commonwealth Games proves it.

Considering his massive successes in lifting, you would think that Dave knew all the answers, and knew that he did, but that's not the way it is at all. In the years that I have known Dave Morgan, he has never stopped reading, asking questions and experimenting; he's ever on the quest to learn more, and to turn that knowledge into better training and competition results.

And this is also the reason I believe *Be Your Best* is one of the most comprehensive and effective fitness books on the market. Whatever your age, shape, size or level of fitness, Dave's simple-to-follow nutrition and training program will achieve fantastic results and set you on the route to optimum health – for life.

So, if you're too skinny, too fat, too weak or just generally in poor physical condition, turn the page and get on a new road . . . *Be Your Best*.

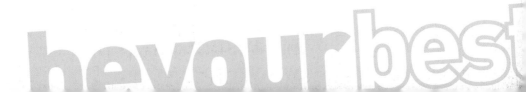

introduction and overview

beyourbest

Hello and welcome to *Be Your Best*.

My name is David Morgan and I have written this book because I wanted to share the most effective way to get into good shape and stay there.

I have been involved in health and fitness for over thirty years and during that time have read hundreds of books, spoken to hundreds of experts (some real and some not) and, more importantly, tried just about everything. And during that time I have learned that you cannot cheat science. Not for long, anyway.

The only real way to get in shape and stay there is to:

1. Adopt correct eating habits (that does not mean going on a diet)

2. Use strength training to build and maintain muscle

3. Use cardiovascular (CV) training to build and maintain heart fitness

4. Get enough rest and recovery

I will show you the right way to eat and train for long-term success.

This book contains clear up-to-date information that will motivate you by explaining *why* and *how* smart training and smart eating will give you the best chance of getting and staying fit and healthy.

Smart eating and smart training are not about quick ways to diet or get fit; they're about taking responsibility for your own good health for as long as you can. This book helps you to chart your progress through months and years. The energy you need from food, the way you exercise to burn it and the results you get depend on what you want to achieve, your body type and your starting point.

These things change, and my Rotational and Progressive system will show you how to balance and vary your exercise and eating regime.

If the life you lead makes you feel physically mediocre . . .
I'll show you how to live at your optimum level of fitness for the rest of your life.

Remember how exhilarating running and jumping was when you were young? Healthy children are always active, building muscle and using up energy from morning until night. But take a look around you. Thirty years on, most of the population are pretty out of condition. What happened to all that limitless energy?

Somewhere along the line, people get out of practice. They eat and drink the wrong things, drive everywhere, take no exercise. They don't manage their time well enough.

But let me put your mind at rest by telling you that it's never too late. You *can* get that energy back.

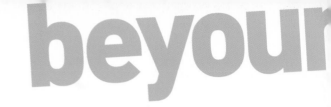

If you already train, feel good, and want to feel better . . .

As everybody knows, most people stop going to the gym because they expect instant results and are discouraged by the amount of work involved. Others, sometimes people who've been training for a few years, slowly wind down because they get bored and frustrated.

They reach a plateau and can't go beyond it, or their circumstances change and they don't make time for the weekly training that turns feeling more-or-less OK into feeling on top of the world. These are just blips in your fitness – unless you let yourself slide out of the training habit for good. You can't afford the luxury of a sedentary life. And don't make the mistake of thinking that age alone is any reason to stop. If you need proof, watch any big marathon and you'll see runners in their seventh, eighth and even ninth decade.

If you're seriously overweight, this book can help . . .

As I write, the official statistics show that a horrifying 40 per cent of the population in the UK is overweight. Of this percentage just over half are considered clinically obese.

This is sad because being overweight affects your general health and longevity and, of course, your family life. What's worse is that if you keep making bad choices, eating and drinking the wrong things and gain only a few pounds a year – well, you can work out for yourself how long it'll take you to become that overweight, lethargic person – and, once you reach that stage, it gets harder for your younger energetic self to break out.

If you follow the advice this book gives you, you will lose fat and simultaneously gain cardiovascular fitness, strength and muscle tone, along with the confidence to want to keep training and a tremendous sense of achievement.

Heard it all before?

Health and fitness is an industry. It is selling something.

This means two things: first, it's not going to tell you any bad news; second, it has got to keep interesting you in new products.

It can give you some awesome opportunities, though. All you do is fill in your credit card number, unpack the biodynamically engineered rowing machine as soon as it's delivered, and you'll have an iron-hard stomach and muscular limbs in just ten days. And because of your hectic lifestyle, you really should take a new supplement made from the pollen of Japanese bindweed.

Yes, the industry does sell snake oil. And it is confusing, and it is worth a whole lot of money. But all over the world there are centenarians enjoying life – as fit as fleas; some are still working. Without exception, these people eat delicious healthy food and stay active all day long. So far as scientists can tell, their genetic inheritance is only a small part of it. Diet, exercise and constant

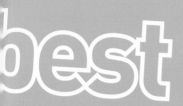
best

challenges are key factors in promoting mental, as well as physical, longevity.

There's one other thing. It's becoming increasingly clear that optimism makes a difference - which in turn is affected by physical wellbeing.

So at the bottom of the health and fitness industry is one sound message: *You can be your best for longer than you think.*

what's wrong with diets?

There are hundreds of fad diets and fad exercise regimes on the market, but they never last - have you ever asked yourself why? Because none of them works long term!

Sure, you can restrict your carbohydrates and lose ten pounds in a week, but most of that weight loss will be through dehydration, not fat loss. You will also feel awful because you are cutting out something vital that your body really needs. This type of 'diet' also makes your body release certain chemicals - which can make you smell bad!

This kind of weight loss is an illusion, a quick fix designed to trick you into thinking that you are being successful.

There is no secret diet or exercise machine that will get you into shape in weeks with no effort, so you're wasting your time by looking for it.

The sad thing is that virtual starvation diets and endless aerobic training will work in the short term. Unfortunately the long-term result of this regime is that you will eventually turn your body into a fat-gaining machine. This is the opposite of what you were trying to achieve. How ironic is that?

Let me explain.

Starvation diets do not give your body the nutrients that it needs. Therefore, two things happen:

1. You eventually go back to your original eating regime

2. You lose valuable fat-burning muscle

Add endless aerobic training to the mix and you accelerate the muscle-loss process.

Why is it so important to keep your muscle?
Muscle is living tissue. It's what enables us to move and because it is living tissue it uses up energy. So the more you have the more calories you will burn. Start losing it and you will burn fewer calories and become more susceptible to fat gain. Muscle also has other benefits. It makes us strong and shapes our bodies.

why bother?

Maintain a smart-eating and smart-training regime and you'll be at your best. You'll be a happy, confident person because you're doing yourself justice. You may be thinking that smart training sounds like hard work. It can be sometimes, especially if you haven't tried it before. Like any new discipline, whether it's learning a language or finding out how to use a computer, there's a steeper learning curve at the start. As you train harder, developing muscles may make you a bit sore after training at first. Later on, when you understand that you're not hurting yourself but helping, stamina may be a challenge.

But habit kicks in; you learn to incorporate regular exercise and training into your life, so it becomes unthinkable not to go to the gym or train regularly, because you'd feel bad. You'd feel uneasy, somehow at odds with the way you usually are, like someone who's left the house without cleaning their teeth.

As for eating - perhaps you think smart eating means rabbit food. Well, I have never eaten rabbit food and I don't intend to start. Eating healthily is not 'unfashionable' and can also be enjoyable. Eating healthily has been normal for most people the world over throughout history and still is. Fresh unprocessed food and drink, produced as close to home as possible, is normal.

What is dysfunctional, in dietary terms, is the kind of processed food that was necessary to feed all the millions who flooded into cities throughout the industrial revolution, but isn't necessary to anyone shopping today. What is dysfunctional is the addictive overuse of

fats, sugar and salt, which manufacturers use to get you hooked and bulk out their product cheaply. Nothing could be more of a false economy.

If you eat healthily you won't gain weight and you will gradually lose any unnatural cravings you ever had for fat, sugar or salt. If you learn to eat healthily, you don't even think about chips and sweets; you just reject junk and enjoy discovering the endless variety of delicious flavours and textures in real food.

Combine smart eating with smart training, and you will see measurable progress. You will build muscle, reduce fat and your lung capacity will improve. You will also be more mentally alert. As you move into middle and old age, you will remain strong and active.

Better things to do with my time . . .
Really? Name one. And tell me you wouldn't do it better if you were in better shape.

real life

I do understand that there are times when you will miss a training session or will eat out and spoil yourself. I have been training since I was twelve, and I'm still making improvements - although I very rarely miss a training session, I do indulge from time to time and satisfy my sweet tooth. But I don't beat myself up over it or dwell on feeling guilty. Success is about what you do most of the time; so, as long as you follow the principles and plans in this book most of the time, the odd slip or moment of indulgence won't matter in the long run.

1

what do you want to achieve?

beyourbest

Look at your personal goals with a steely eye.
Be realistic: don't set yourself up to fail. If anyone
tells you a treadmill or a weight-loss diet will give
you the perfect body in weeks, react with Jeremy
Paxman-like scepticism.

Yes, it takes time. And you need a personal goal you can reach, not one that is – if you're starting from a very low base – way, way over the horizon. The good news is that most goals are attainable with a well-structured eating plan and two to three hours of training every week; but you have to get there step by step, and the more ambitious the goal, the longer it takes.

In the next chapter, you can define your situation in detail: where, in physical terms, you are now, and where you want your fitness programme to take you. You'll define exactly how you'd like your body to improve. You may want to lose fat, gain muscle, get stronger or just improve your general aerobic fitness.

You may train regularly already, but find yourself at a frustrating plateau. If this is so, shift focus. Following the Rotational and Progressive four-step system (see page 97) will help you refocus and move past your sticking point. This book teaches you a system that allows you to continue to improve. It also explains the importance of rest and recovery and how changes of diet can have a positive impact on your life.

You may want to maintain general all-round fitness while continuing to improve your strength and muscle tone.

I rotate my training regime. I start by focusing on general fitness; then on strength and muscle gain and then fat loss. The Rotational and Progressive system is based on this approach. What I want you

beyourbest

to understand is that being your best isn't about just one thing – it's about integrating many activities and attitudes into your life. But the one that most concerns most people who feel less than their best is fat loss.

fat loss

Being overweight is a big problem in America and the UK (we're the fattest people in Europe) because of our fondness for processed food and alcohol. The way our cities and towns are designed doesn't help either; there's a built-in disincentive to walking anywhere.

You are statistically extremely unlikely to lose fat permanently on a 'diet'. Nor will you lose it by just exercising.

To see excess fat come off and never return, you need to establish and maintain a structured exercise plan whilst eating healthily: daily and for life. This is not a diet but a change of lifestyle. A healthier lifestyle means leaving the car at home whenever you can, and smart eating and drinking: as little processed food as possible, and alcohol occasionally rather than every night.

The reasons are simple. Exercise strengthens your muscles and bones and makes you happier, which in turn makes you more energetic and more attractive. Refusing processed food inevitably means eating more fibre and less sugar, salt and saturated fat. Refusing alcohol means you're not pouring useless calories into your overburdened frame, but liberating your midriff.

Remember: this is a journey. If you are obese, rather than slightly overweight, there is absolutely no point in going hell-for-leather in the gym; you won't enjoy yourself and you will risk injury. My Rotational and Progressive approach is suitable for anyone. You start by eating properly and building regular exercise into your daily routine. You need to understand your starting point and build from it slowly.

There is a lot more in Chapter 4 (Smart Eating) about food, drink and nutrition.

muscle gain

Your body will be some variant on one of the three basic body types. These are called somatotypes: ectomorphic, endomorphic and mesomorphic. Ectomorphs are skinny and often tall. They find it hard to gain fat easily, which is not a bad thing, but they don't gain much muscle easily either. Endomorphs build up both: they can have arms like pistons and a beer belly. Mesomorphs are the athletic ideal since they store fat at a manageable rate but build muscle quite quickly.

Regardless of your somatotype, you can shape and improve your body and fitness levels. With progressive training, attention to diet and adequate protein, your body can lose fat and gain muscle in the right places and start to look the way you want it to.

Do you think you're just flabby, rather than fat? If so, you need to aim to lose excess fat and gain muscle at the same time: this will give your body better definition. Or you may be skinny, in which case you will gain muscle more efficiently if you eat properly and train more intensely but not so often. Most people can put on two to five kilos (about five to eleven pounds) of muscle in a year. Read the Smart Eating chapter to find out about eating for measured energy release throughout the day, fat loss and muscle gain. Chapter 9 shows the changes you need to make to your diet depending on your specific goal.

getting stronger

You don't need to be a particular genetic type to be strong. In my experience, the average person can easily double their strength over time with a few hours' regular weekly training. Some individuals have the potential to increase their strength by up to 400 per cent.

Just to put strength into perspective, if you can do forty press-ups, you're in the top 10 per cent of the population. If you can bench-press your own bodyweight for ten reps, you're in the top 1 per cent.

And if you are mystified by exactly how to do a bench press or what a bench press is, don't worry. Chapter 7 explains how to use equipment and how to do all the exercises.

get fitter

If you want all-round fitness you must do some aerobic exercise because aerobic fitness relates to the heart and lungs that keep you going. Exercise of almost any kind (flicking the remote control doesn't count) increases the supply of oxygen in your blood, which keeps your brain alert and your muscles primed for action.

If you are overweight and over forty, look on the bright side: you already have what they call 'away from' motivation to get aerobically fitter. You're getting 'away from' the likelihood that you may get type-2 diabetes and be at higher risk of stroke, heart disease and certain cancers. The minute you start, you've taken a decisive step away from all that. Take the PAR Q test (in Chapter 2) before you start your exercise regime.

And if you smoke at any age, you'll be exercising at less than your full lung capacity, which means you have to work harder to get results. Even if your body shape improves, it is impossible to be your best as a smoker.

Cut down and stop; you'll feel better and have more money, more opportunities and better teeth.

If you want all-round fitness you must do some aerobic exercise because aerobic fitness relates to the heart and lungs that keep you going. Exercise of almost any kind (flicking the remote control doesn't count) increases the supply of oxygen in your blood, which keeps your brain alert and your muscles primed for action.

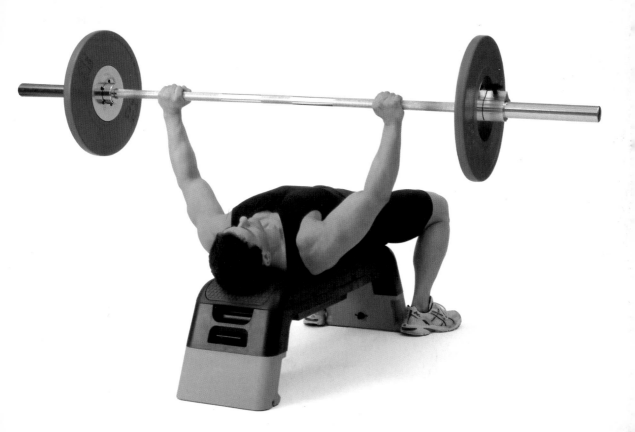

beyourbest

motivation

Like most achievers, I believe in goal setting but I also believe in rest and rewards. I think of smart training as a lifelong challenge rather than a series of deadlines based on time.

Getting anything done to a deadline is fine but, if you've also got to reach a new personal best within a deadline, it can be stressful. Concentrate on good daily habits and being your best will just happen. Your goal is to keep working towards what you want to achieve. It will take some people longer than others for all sorts of reasons. Remember, it's not a race – it's establishing lifestyle changes that incrementally enable you to move towards better health and fitness, and a better life.

Establish good habits, and your occasional 'indulgence' will be doubly enjoyable and won't stunt your progress.

Most people make the effort to look their best when they get married or go on holiday, because people take a lot of notice of the way you look at times like that. Besides, the photographs will be there for your grandchildren to laugh at, so you'd better get your act together.

By the time you've read this book you'll be realistic about the targets you can reach in the time you're willing to make available. More importantly, I hope you'll like your new lifestyle and your new, better-looking self well enough to carry on improving.

My approach to training is designed to help you meet your health and fitness objectives and become your best – for life. That applies whoever you are, whatever your goals and whatever your starting point.

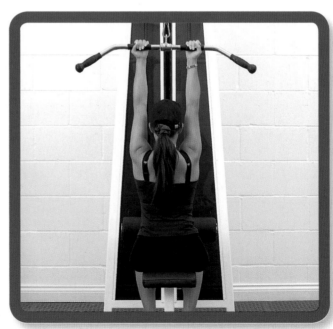

2

where are you now?

> **Your aim is to be your best, so, to motivate yourself and work towards your goals, you'll need to fill in a record book religiously at every stage.**

First, establish your starting point - the present relationship of fat to muscle in your body, how fit you are, your feelings about exercise generally and the factors likely to be affected by your age, lifestyle and motivation. You will need:

 A tape measure

 Accurate bathroom scales (use the same scales on the same type of floor for consistency every time you weigh yourself)

 A camera, preferably set to print the date on your pictures

 A record book - a hard-backed A4 notebook in which to record your results: date, weight, measurements and achievements

Now you've decided to start, take it for granted that you'll still be keeping track of progress when you're 95. You can be your best for life - one goal achieved will lead to the next.

your start weight

Your weight doesn't necessarily indicate whether or not you're 'overweight'. For a true picture you need to know how much muscle you have in relation to fat.

However, you do need to write down your bodyweight at the beginning because it is important to the overall picture, so weigh yourself accurately one morning, naked and before breakfast. Allow at least a week between weigh-ins and always weigh yourself at the same time; you are generally heavier in the evening because of the food and drink you've consumed during the course of the day.

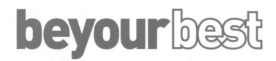

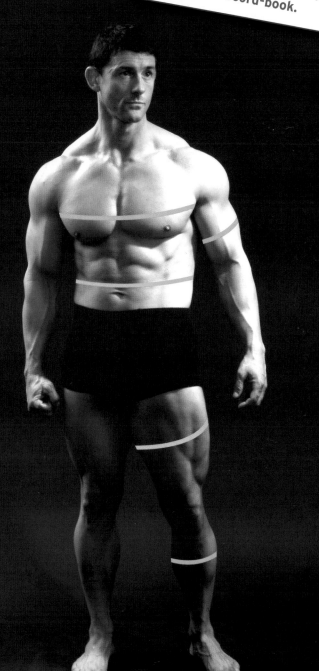

your start
measurements

Measure your waist, chest and limbs as indicated in the picture, and note the results under today's date in your record-book.

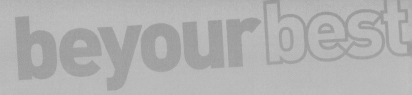

Suppose that three months after you start smart eating and smart training, you find you've gained five pounds. If those five pounds on the scales are accompanied by a three-inch loss around your waist, then you've gained muscle and lost fat. Your trousers will feel looser around the waist and you'll look better than you did in your start photographs.

You're achieving results – and your measurements, combined with your bodyweight, your training results and the way you feel, will prove it.

your start bmi and w2w

You now need to calculate how much fat you're carrying around. Your BMI (body mass index) is a rough guide popular with doctors; it doesn't measure muscle-to-fat ratio, but does indicate whether you're overweight or clinically obese in relation to your height and population averages. Many top athletes would be overweight on the BMI scale, because of the extra muscle they carry.

If you haven't taken much exercise for months or years the BMI may have some relevance. Check your BMI using the calculation below and then use the chart to see which range you fall into: obese, overweight, within the 'normal' range or underweight.

bmi calculation

BMI = weight in kilos divided by height in metres squared

So, someone 1.72m (5ft 8in) tall weighing 85kg (187lb) would have the following BMI:

BMI = 85 / (1.72 x 1.72) = 85 / 2.9584 = 28.7

To convert:
cm to inches   *divide by 2.54*
inches to cm   *multiply by 2.54*
kg to lb   *multiply by 2.2*
lb to kg   *divide by 2.2*

To analyse your results see the chart below:

bmi	weight status
Below 18.5	Underweight
18.5-24.9	Normal
25.0-29.9	Overweight
30.0 and above	Obese

If you do train regularly you may have built enough muscle to make the BMI test irrelevant. In this situation, the W2W (waist to weight) calculation is going to be more suitable.

It is an easy-to-use and reasonably accurate way to measure the proportion of fat you're carrying around in relation to your weight. Check your weight against your waist measurement in the following chart.

You now need to calculate how much fat you're carrying around. Your BMI (body mass index) is a rough guide popular with doctors

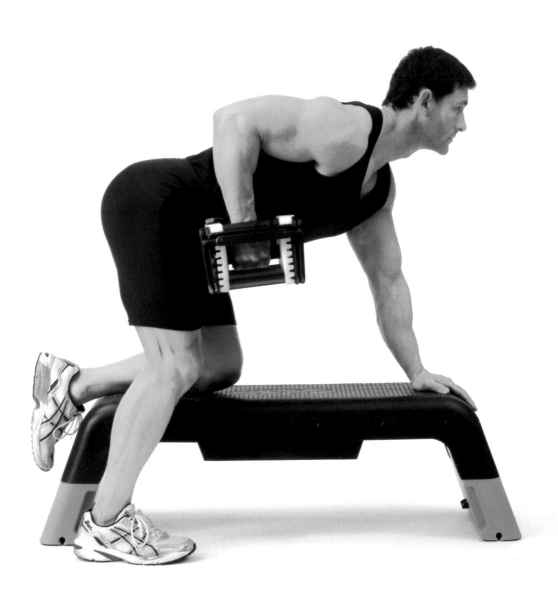

Because women tend to carry less muscle than men, the BMI is more accurate, while, for men, the W2W is better.

w2w chart

In the chart below, find your weight in the left-hand column and your waist measurement in the right-hand column. Draw a straight line between the two measurements and where the line crosses the middle column (percent fat) will give you an indication of your body fat percentage. The table below the chart shows the body fat percentage ranges and the categories they are associated with.

classification	% fat
Essential fat	2-4%
Athletes	6-13%
Fitness	14-17%
Acceptable	18-25%
Obese	25% plus

your start photographs

Take three photographs. One is full frontal, one from the side and one from the back. (Sense dictates that you will wear shorts for these, unless you want to risk flashing around the world by mobile phone.)

Waist (inches)

Body weight (kg)

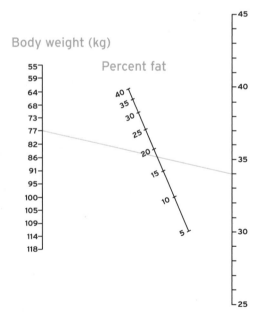

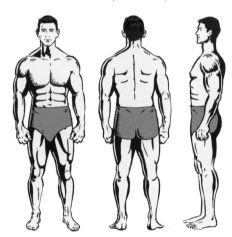

Take them against a plain background in good light, somewhere you can revisit to shoot fresh pictures three to six months from now. You need consistent points of comparison if you're to get a true measure of your progress. Date them and keep them with your record book.

absolute beginners

Before you start an exercise programme you should answer some basic questions called the PAR Q (Physical Activity Readiness Questions). For each question below, tick the box that applies to you.

Yes No

☐ ☐ Has your doctor ever said you have heart trouble?

☐ ☐ Do you frequently have pains in your heart and chest?

☐ ☐ Do you often feel faint or have dizzy spells?

☐ ☐ Has a doctor ever said your blood pressure was too high?

☐ ☐ Has your doctor ever told you that you have a bone or joint problem such as arthritis that has been aggravated by exercise, or might worsen with exercise?

☐ ☐ Is there any other good physical reason why you should not follow an activity programme?

☐ ☐ Are you over 65 and not used to vigorous exercise?

Take medical advice if you answer yes to any of the above questions.

If you answer no to all the questions, you can go ahead and take a basic fitness test.

The two illustrated below are the Step Test, which gauges your aerobic heart and lung capacity, and the Press-up Test, to find your strength level.

3-minute step test

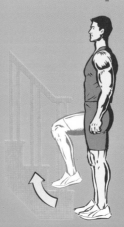

This test is designed to measure your cardiovascular endurance. Using a twelve-inch-high bench (or a similar-sized stair in your house), step on and off for three minutes. Step up with one foot and then the other. Step down with one foot followed by the other foot. Try to maintain a steady four-beat cycle – it's easy to maintain if you say 'up, up, down, down'. Go at a steady and consistent pace.

At the end of three minutes, remain standing while you immediately check your heart rate by taking your pulse for one minute. Compare your result to the chart on the following page.

For a more accurate text you can find details on my website www.beyourbest-davidmorgan.com

How did you do? look at the table below and find the column for your age range. Then find your heart rate in the figures in the table for an indication of your fitness.

men

age	18–25	26–35	36–45	46–55	56–65	65+
Excellent	<79	<81	<83	<87	<86	<88
Good	79-89	81-89	83-96	87-97	86-97	88-96
Above Average	90-99	90-99	97-103	98-105	98-103	97-103
Average	100-105	100-107	104-112	106-116	104-112	104-113
Below Average	106-116	108-117	113-119	117-122	113-120	114-120
Poor	117-128	118-128	120-130	123-132	121-129	121-130
Very Poor	>128	>128	>130	>132	>129	>130

women

age	18–25	26–35	36–45	46–55	56–65	65+
Excellent	<85	<88	<90	<94	<95	<90
Good	85-98	88-99	90-102	94-104	95-104	90-102
Above Average	99-108	100-111	103-110	105-115	105-112	103-115
Average	109-117	112-119	111-118	116-120	113-118	116-122
Below Average	118-126	120-126	119-128	121-129	119-128	123-128
Poor	127-140	127-138	129-140	130-135	129-139	129-134
Very Poor	>140	>138	>140	>135	>139	>134

how to take your heart rate

Your heart rate can be taken at any spot on the body where an artery is close to the surface and a pulse can be felt. The most common places to measure heart rate using the palpation method are at the wrist and the neck. Other places sometimes used are the elbow and the groin.

To take your resting heart rate at the wrist, place your index and middle fingers together on the opposite wrist, about half an inch from the inside of the joint, in line with the index finger. Feel for a pulse and, when you find one, count the number of beats you feel within a one-minute period. You can estimate the per-minute rate by counting over 10 seconds and multiplying this figure by 6, or over 15 seconds and multiplying by 4, or over 30 seconds and doubling the result. (There are obvious potential errors by using this shorthand method.)

You should always use your fingers to take a pulse, not your thumb, particularly when recording someone else's pulse, as you can sometimes feel your own pulse through your thumb.

press-up test

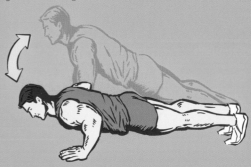

How many press-ups can you do? Use the standard 'military-style' press-up position with only the hands and the toes touching the floor. Women have the option of using the 'bent-knee' position. To do this, kneel on the floor, hands on either side of the chest, and keep your back straight. Do as many press-ups as possible until exhaustion. Count the total number performed and use the charts below and on the following page to find out how you rate.

men

age	17–19	20–29	30–39	40–49	50–59	60–65
Excellent	>56	>47	>41	>34	>31	>30
Good	47-56	39-47	34-41	28-34	25-31	24-30
Above average	35-46	30-39	25-33	21-28	18-24	17-23
Average	19-34	17-29	13-24	11-20	9-17	6-16
Below average	11-18	10-16	8-12	6-10	5-8	3-5
Poor	4-10	4-9	2-7	1-5	1-4	1-2
Very Poor	<4	<4	<2	0	0	0

women

Age	17–19	20–29	30–39	40–49	50–59	60–65
Excellent	>35	>36	>37	>31	>25	>23
Good	27-35	30-36	30-37	25-31	21-25	19-23
Above Average	21-27	23-29	22-30	18-24	15-20	13-18
Average	11-20	12-22	10-21	8-17	7-14	5-12
Below average	6-10	7-11	5-9	4-7	3-6	2-4
Poor	2-5	2-6	1-4	1-3	1-2	1
Very Poor	0-1	0-1	0	0	0	0

Please note these tests are just meant as a basic guide to give you a point of reference to start from.

your points of departure

You've now established your physical starting point for smart eating and smart training. Even if you're already going to the gym regularly, it's no bad idea to revisit this chapter because it may remind you of why you started and what your own strengths and weaknesses are.

Step back and assess other things besides your physical condition. You're not doing this for a quick fix, so set up a routine that suits you.

First of all, timing: if you go home from work on a cold January night, fully intending to go to the gym later, you probably won't. But, if you arrange regular workouts before you start work or before you go home, training integrates seamlessly into your day.

And frequency: you don't need to train every lunchtime and after work – in fact, you shouldn't. Anyone who isn't preparing for the Olympics and finds that training leaves no time for a social life is taking themselves too seriously. Two to three hours a week are enough. (If you work eighteen-hour days and have 'no time', for training or anything else, then you, more than anyone, need to be at your physical best – so it might be time for a rethink.)

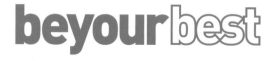

And flexibility: accept that your training routine will adjust when your life changes direction. Be prepared to readjust - but not to stop - your gym habit when you move house or change job. If you are ill you should not train until fully recovered.

Perhaps you've trained before and you didn't think you were getting anywhere? I would doubt whether you were measuring your progress accurately or following a progressive plan. Always, always keep your record book. With training, improvement is measurable and your record book is the best motivator you'll ever have.

your pbs

Your Personal Bests - your best 2000-metre rowing time or best bench press for ten repetitions, for instance - are great motivators.

I often work with people who've been training at gyms alone, some of them for many years. I ask them what their personal records are and I am surprised by the number who have no idea.

Knowledge is power. If you're running a business, you naturally keep a record of what sales promotions work (or don't) and what sells and what doesn't. The most successful businesses are the ones that are totally on top of every detail and use what they know as a tool to improve performance. It's the same with training: don't waste time and effort, but observe and record, and make your observations work for you. Sometimes you'll reach a plateau, and your key to reaching the next level may be something as minor as an extra repetition, an extra set, a slight change of diet or more rest. You won't know, unless you've kept detailed records, exactly what your key to improvement might be.

Another thing that successful businesses - and individuals - do is set goals and visualise achievement. In the course of your active life you'll set many short-term goals, and with persistence they will always be reached. Success isn't a destination - it's a journey. Keep track of your route!

at my age . . .

This book is called *Be Your Best* for a reason and provides anyone of any age with a plan that works.

There are some events - the extraordinarily gruelling Tour de France is one - where the most successful athletes tend to be over thirty. And you're never too old to see real improvement even if you've never taken much exercise.

In his eightieth year, my friend's father Ron has a medical history that includes a broken neck, arthritis and, just recently, a knee replacement. He was due to go into hospital to get the other knee replaced, but wanted to strengthen both legs first.

He passed all his general health tests, so we began to experiment with different leg exercises. Some were impossible for him, because of his dodgy knee, but there were plenty of others to try. He found he could use the leg press without pain, so that's where we started. We also added upper-body movements. These gave variety to each session and balance to the training regime, and meant he had more opportunities to improve, succeed and feel good – positive reinforcement in every way. I wanted these sessions to be enjoyable, so that after recovery from the operation Ron would come back.

I always knew the result would be good, but I admit to astonishment when in three months he increased his leg press PB from 20kg (44lb) for 20 reps, to 240kg (528lb) for 20 reps and he had increased his range of movement as well, which meant he could add dead lifts to the programme. Dead lifts work the whole body together, and as a result he is able to walk with more confidence. His balance has improved and he has doubled his upper-body strength.

Ron's recovery from his first knee operation had taken six months, but this time it took only three.

Ron had a clear idea of what he wanted to achieve, and consistently recorded his training and his personal bests. He still does. He's a regular at the gym and continues to make great gains. He says that, because he feels stronger, he feels good about himself and his quality of life has improved a lot. He's walking better than ever with the new knee and is much better able to cope with the arthritis.

Exercise helps brain and body at any age: it's a fact. That should be a motivating factor for all of us.

Remember: Strength training combined with aerobic work, good nutrition and adequate rest for recovery are the keys to long-term health and fitness.

3

still need
convincing?

> **This chapter of horror and negativity is for everyone who lives by the following formula:**
> **no exercise + junk food + smoking + excessive drinking = healthy enough**

why gamble?

Nothing great ever got done without somebody, somewhere, taking a risk. But there's a big difference between risk - which is an informed, calculated chance taken for a worthwhile reward - and a gamble. A gamble is by definition entirely reliant on luck and the chances are always stacked against you.

If your lifestyle matches the above formula you are taking a gamble. You may well feel fine in your twenties, thirties and forties. Meanwhile, out of sight and out of mind, the diseases caused by living like this are inexorably developing in your bloodstream and internal organs. Twenty years on, when you're being wheeled in for a triple bypass, you may regret the self-neglect that presented itself as self-indulgence at the time.

In fact, no exercise + junk food + excessive drinking = lower likelihood of staying healthy enough to enjoy life after fifty. If you smoke heavily and do other social drugs as well, then the odds are mounting up, but not in your favour.

Maybe you live by the maxim, **'You've got to die of something . . .'**

If you are already overweight, eat junk, smoke, take no exercise and drink too much, you have probably forgotten how it feels to be really healthy and are probably just used to feeling 'crap' all the time.

Running your body on pizza, ice cream and beer is like trying to run a Mercedes on cooking oil. You fur up, slow down and end up parked in life's garage - inactive, with low self-esteem. After that it's just a roll off the couch before you meet type-2 diabetes, stroke, heart disease, gallstones, incontinence, osteoarthritis, sleep apnoea or one of the many cancers that you are at high risk of getting if you don't eat and drink healthily and take exercise.

Still think you've got to die of something?

Read on.

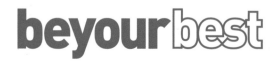

heart disease and cardiovascular disease

Heart disease is what it says. Cardiovascular disease, on the other hand, affects not only the heart, but the entire circulatory system that drives blood through your torso, limbs and brain. Your blood-pressure reading is a measure of the force with which blood is being pumped. When the nurse mutters '120 over 80' as she removes the band from your arm, she means that the systolic pressure (of oxygenated, nutrient-rich blood pumping out through the arteries to make your body work) is 120 and the diastolic pressure (of depleted blood flowing back through the veins) is 80. If the reading is 140 over 90 or above, you have high blood pressure and your heart is struggling to pump the blood through arteries that may be damaged or partly blocked. You are at higher risk of heart attack or stroke and a number of other complications – for instance with your kidneys and eyes – related to your heart and blood flow.

You don't know you've got high blood pressure until you test it, and for regular check-ups you can buy a testing kit at the chemist's.

Then there's a heart attack. You may feel pain or a sort of squeezing feeling in the centre of your chest that goes on for a few minutes, or comes and goes. The pains may seem to spread to your arms or jaw or stomach, and you can get cold sweats and want to be sick. You will be very scared and so will those around you.

With long-term cardiovascular disease, the arteries often develop aneurisms – little bulges in the blood vessels – or fur up with something entirely avoidable, called plaque, causing sluggish blood flow all round. Symptoms include breathlessness, confusion, worsening eyesight, kidney problems and sometimes fluid retention. You may have a heart attack or a stroke.

lifestyle risk factors

Smoking: Smokers are up to four times more likely to get heart disease than nonsmokers, and twice as likely to die of a sudden heart attack.

Eating lots of butter, hard cheese and fatty red meat: High blood cholesterol is usually the result, along with too much LDL cholesterol, which furs up arteries.

Physical inactivity: Blood pressure is lowered to a healthy level by regular brisk exercise.

Eating salty food: Too much salt retained in the blood causes its volume to increase and your blood pressure to rise. Your heart has to work harder to pump the blood around, causing strain on the artery walls, which can make them thicken and harden.

Obesity and being overweight: Carrying fat around the waist dramatically increases your risk of developing heart disease.

Diabetes: Too much refined sugar makes you a candidate for type-2 diabetes. Diabetes seriously increases your risk of a heart attack, even when blood-glucose levels are under control and particularly when they are not. Three-quarters of people with diabetes die of some form of heart or cardiovascular disease.

Alcohol: Drinking more than the recommended limit can lead to high blood pressure and heart failure, not to mention kidney and liver problems. Excessive drinking is also closely linked to being overweight because of the high calorie content in alcohol.

stroke

A stroke can be caused by a blockage in the blood flow to the brain, or a burst blood vessel that interrupts blood supply to the brain; so a stroke is a particular kind of cardiovascular disease. As a result of even a minor stroke, brain cells immediately die. It is the third biggest killer after heart disease and cancer: every three minutes, somebody has a stroke, and, although most of them are over 65, many are much younger.

A fatal stroke may or may not be preceded by a minor attack. Suddenly one side of your face, or a leg or an arm, will feel weak or numb. You may feel oddly confused, or have trouble understanding speech or speaking or seeing. You may lose your balance, or suddenly get a bad headache, or feel sleepy or nauseous. All these can indicate that you are having a stroke, from which recovery can be slow and frustrating.

You are at high risk of a stroke if you:

(!) Have high blood pressure (keep the numbers below 120 over 80; 140/90 is high)

(!) Smoke (stop now)

(!) Have a high LDL cholesterol level and a low HDL cholesterol level (keep your LDL level below 3 and your HDL above 1)

(!) Are overweight or obese (check your BMI – see Chapter 2)

(!) Are physically inactive

(!) Have diabetes

(!) Eat and drink unhealthily

(!) Have heart disease

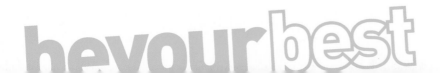

type-2 diabetes

Insulin is a hormone that your pancreas pumps into your blood to regulate the level of sugar in it. When you consume sweet drinks or food, a healthy pancreas pumps out some insulin into the blood so the system isn't overwhelmed with glucose, but regulates its distribution to the organs that need it. Some people are born with a tendency to produce insufficient insulin and their type-1 diabetes is usually diagnosed in childhood; it's regulated by medication that may include insulin injections.

What used to be called late-onset diabetes is now known as type-2, because it isn't late-onset any more. Children as young as ten have developed it as a direct consequence of eating refined sugar in processed foods and drinking sweet soft drinks as a baby. There is an epidemic of type-2 diabetes in parts of New York – and, like much American culture, it's probably coming our way.

A person can abuse their pancreas only so much. If, year after year, it's asked to pump out floods of insulin, several times a day, it will go on strike. You'll start getting highs and lows: sugar rushes, followed by faintness, constant thirst and tiredness. When your pancreas can no longer produce enough insulin to regulate and redistribute your blood sugar you will get type-2 diabetes, and are old before your time.

The disease is a leading cause of blindness. Diabetics have more gum and tooth problems than other people. They have poor circulation in the legs and feet – more than half the amputees in the United States lose their limbs because of diabetes. They are at high risk of kidney dysfunction, heart disease and, of course, diabetic coma.

Type-2 diabetes is certainly preventable with exercise and correct diet, and if caught in its early stages is manageable, but full recovery is unusual.

do you see a pattern?

People *can* drop dead of a heart attack when they are healthy, just as they can smoke like chimneys and survive into their nineties. But not many do – and why gamble with the only life you've got?

People who say 'You've got to die of something' expect to keel over painlessly one day when they're past caring. Death's not like that. Nearly all deaths come as the final act in a chronic disease you'll have lived with for years, which was probably preventable.

If your first fifty years are spent furring up your arteries, letting your muscles waste away and piling on fat, then your last twenty or thirty may be spent in a wheelchair, in and out of hospital, gasping for breath, fearing amputation, having to relearn to talk after a stroke, living with incontinence, and knowing that you will never be able to play in the park with your grandchildren or even get on an aeroplane again.

Grim? Yes, it is. It is the reality of life for millions of older people. If you don't see them, it's because they don't get out much.

Heart attacks, strokes and cancer are the top three killers. A World Health Organisation report in 2005 said 80 per cent of heart disease, stroke and type-2 diabetes and 40 per cent of cancers could be avoided through healthy diet, regular physical activity and avoiding smoking. Diabetes-related deaths are expected to rise by 25 per cent in the UK between 2005 and 2015.

Addiction to cigarettes or alcohol, or consuming too much refined sugar, fatty or salty foods can cause all the diseases in this chapter. Addictions like these are often encouraged, and not just by advertising. There's social pressure to get a lager and a curry and jeers if you choose a lean chicken salad and a glass of water. Alcohol has no nutritional value and is very high in calories. It doesn't help you relax or aid sleep and is closely associated with diabetes and obesity - yet binge drinking is becoming increasingly common.

Too much salt causes damage too. The extent to which each person responds to a high intake of salt is probably genetically determined. Some people are more susceptible to the effects than others, and sensitivity appears to increase with age.

Increased salt intake causes more fluid to be contained in the blood vessels. This increased volume of blood requires the heart to work harder to pump blood to all the tissues in the body. Increasing the blood's volume within the enclosure of the circulatory system is one way that salt increases blood pressure.

It's your life. What you put in your body is your business. You'll be doing yourself, and your family, a favour if you make a lifelong habit of smart eating and smart training.

You'll have the last laugh, too.

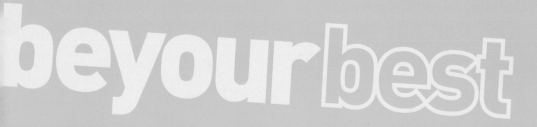

4

smart
eating

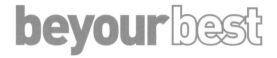

beyourbest

> **Diet (definition): A short-term restriction of calories and necessary nutrients.**

how diets cause trouble

You start dieting in order to lose fat. You restrict calories drastically, and find you've lost weight. Some of that was fat, some was muscle, and – if you've been restricting carbohydrates – a lot of it was water.

So have you succeeded? Of course not. It's great that you've lost the fat. But the muscle loss will make you get fatter again faster. Losing muscle isn't good, and your metabolic rate – the rate at which you burn calories at rest – naturally slows down to compensate. So when you stop dieting you will gain weight more quickly. Your metabolism won't speed up again unless you get your muscle back; but, once muscle has gone, it takes a while to build up again. And it's not just your biceps – it's the muscles that work your internal organs that are depleted by dieting.

If you repeat this cycle over and over, you'll progressively lose more muscle and slow down your metabolism still more, predisposing yourself to become one of those people who say they can't look at a carrot without putting on ten pounds. There is some truth in this.

Overweight people who pile on the pounds although they don't eat a lot are victims of this decreased muscle and slow metabolism cycle. It's called rebound weight gain.

why your fat loss slows down

We all accept that if you eat more calories than you burn you will gain fat and if you eat fewer you will lose it. In practice, your body is a bit more complicated. At first, you will lose weight quickly by restricting your calorie intake. But after a while your metabolic rate will slow and stabilise, and with it your weight loss; which is why people complain that it takes them months to shift the last two or three pounds. This happens because we're animals. Your body doesn't know you've got an expense account and a job with Morgan Stanley; it thinks you're scrambling from rock to rock in a loincloth, wondering where the next fistful of nuts and berries is coming from. It has therefore developed a weight-regulating mechanism that recognises when you're not getting enough fuel, and uses less so that you don't 'peg out'. The more calories you cut, the more your body keeps a tight grip on its fat stores. This brilliant adaptation has evolved so that, if you had to, you could survive for months with no food at all, only water.

It is what kept us all alive before Tesco. It's physically impossible to stay on a very-low-calorie diet and lose weight permanently because your physical defence mechanisms kick in. Also, it's just not good for you.

why are diets bad for you?

Most people feel awful when they are hungry. They feel cross and tired. Also they're inwardly worried that their willpower will fail. In the end it will, which will make them feel bad about themselves, which will make them think they are 'weak-willed', which will make them more likely to fail next time.

So, self-loathing aside, what's the case against very-low-calorie diets?

● They deplete muscle, which slows your metabolic rate and leads to rebound weight gain

● They can lead to malnutrition

● They can increase cravings

● They reduce your energy levels and ability to exercise

There is a whole low-protein, high-aerobic-exercise diet fad, mainly popular with girls, but men try it too. Be under no illusions; low-calorie diets with insufficient protein, combined with endless aerobic exercise, cause muscle loss, slower metabolic rate and the need to eat even less and sweat even more in order to stay slim. It's a vicious circle that can ultimately only make you a fatter skinny person.

Diets don't work.

be your best

habits are for life

Long-term success requires smart eating combined with smart training: a permanent change in lifestyle. Forget dieting. Good habits will keep you slim and healthy for life, and you'll never have to worry about your weight.

A habit is something you do automatically, hardly thinking about it. The easiest way to get rid of a bad habit (like dieting) that doesn't work well is to replace it with a new one (like smart eating and smart training) that does.

Good nutritional and exercise habits are as easy to form as bad ones and, once you've formed them, they're just as hard to break. Once you've taught your brain to carry out a certain task in a certain way, it will insist that you keep doing things that way; it's the way our minds work, and a very economical use of brainpower it is too. But our minds are also good at relearning, helping to correct our mistakes and perform tasks even better. By imposing good habits of good nutrition and exercise on yourself, you'll kick out the old ways quite quickly.

It's important to commit yourself 100 per cent from the start. Once the first few weeks of unfamiliar food and exercise have passed, you'll be leaner, fitter and well on your way to being your best – and your new habits will be as effortless and natural as brushing your teeth or taking a shower.

why do i need to exercise as well as eat healthily?

- Exercise – especially weight training – raises your metabolic rate

- Exercise burns fat without causing rebound weight gain

- Exercise is good for you – dieting isn't

- Exercise – especially weight training – tells your body to maintain or build your muscle, not consume it

- Exercise helps your body to burn calories more efficiently; in other words, you become more like one of those people who 'don't put on weight'

why do i need to eat healthily as well as exercise?

Or, why bother with healthy food if I'm going to burn off the calories anyway?

Exercise alone is not enough to keep you fit and healthy. If you are training regularly, it's easy to get complacent about your diet. You can live largely on pork pies and beer, and, as long as you are a nineteen-year-old cycle courier, you'll burn off the calories and still look good – until you get a job in an office and start driving to work. Maybe you have met men in middle age, with paunches and flabby arms, who claim once to have been prop forwards. Where, then, did it all go wrong?

Changes in your daily routine are inevitable, but a healthy diet can be adapted to them so easily that you'll hardly notice. A diet of processed food, on the other hand, cannot be adapted to suit a more sedentary life. It contains too many additives, too much fat, sugar and salt, and too little nutritional value. Its energy is released too quickly into your bloodstream, so it makes you prone to mood swings and fluctuating levels of energy.

the smart eating principles

The principles of smart eating don't change. You will need to alter the emphasis according to whether you're trying to gain muscle, maintain your strength or lose fat; but if you apply the basic principles you'll always eat the best - quality food that will give you the best chance of staying healthy and fit for as long as possible.

These are the principles:

- Choose food in its most natural (unprocessed) state

- Have five meals per day (three main meals containing protein and unrefined carbohydrate and two snacks)

- Make sure there's a little good fat in at least one meal

- And drink plenty of water

not hard, is it?

But, if it were that easy, there wouldn't be one billion obese people in the world. Therefore, it follows that the basic principles need some elaboration.

the food groups and what they do

protein

If you are trying hard to maintain or build muscle and lose fat, it's particularly important to include protein at every meal. Protein helps your muscles develop and repair themselves after exertion. It also slows down the rate at which carbohydrates are released as energy into your body, so it stops you feeling hungry and overeating. Eat a portion with every meal.

carbohydrate

Your body turns carbohydrates into blood sugars for immediate energy. There are four different categories and they are not all good for you.

Complex carbohydrates
These are things like oats, whole grains, wholemeal bread, wholemeal pasta, and rice and root vegetables - including, of course, potatoes. All these come complete with important minerals, vitamins and fibre. The starch converts at a manageable rate into blood sugar for energy, and the roughage helps your digestion. Eat complex carbohydrate early in the day.

The same goes for pulses (beans and lentils); they are useful high-protein carbohydrates.

Simple carbohydrates

These include fruit and are healthy in small quantities. They're fast acting but high in fibre and vitamins. Eat them early in the day, too.

Fibrous carbohydrates

These are green leafy vegetables and salads. They take a long time to digest and are high in nutritional value but low in calories. Eat them with at least two of your daily meals.

Refined carbohydrates

Carbohydrates per se do not make you fat. Refined carbohydrates do. They are calorie-dense, so it is easy for you to eat too many calories. These are things like white sugar (refined out of sugar cane), white flour, white rice, cornflour (refined out of whole grains) and soft drinks. Don't eat or drink any of these. The process of refining removes the fibre and nutritional value (sometimes, as with white flour, to such an extent that the law insists some of the minerals be replaced by the manufacturer).

Read the labels of processed food and you will see that there is sucrose or dextrose or glucose in almost everything. They add bulk cheaply, and make you want to eat more.

Food labelling – do not be fooled by misleading information!

If you are going to get control of your eating you will need to understand what food labels really mean. One of the most misleading pieces of information is fat percentage on packaged foods. All food manufacturers give you the fat percentage of food in grams of fat per 100 grams.

For example, if a food has 10g of fat per 100g it will be labelled as 10 per cent fat. On the face of it this seems logical until you realise that fat grams have 9 calories per gram, whereas protein and carbohydrates only have 4 calories per gram.

This means that, if a product contains a total of 480 calories per 100g and 20 of those grams come from fat, using the grams argument this product would be considered 20 per cent fat.

However, if we calculate by calories, we can see that in fact the product contains 37.5 per cent fat. Let's look at how we arrived at this figure:

Total calories per 100g = 480

Product contains 20g fat, so 20 x 9 calories per gram = 180 calories

So the fat percentage = (180 / 480) x 100 = 0.375 x 100 = 37.5%

As a rough guide the fat percentage of all foods is about double the stated grams per 100 grams. So anything listed as 10 per cent fat by grams is actually about 20 per cent fat by calories.

Avoid heavily processed foods. Most of them, from breakfast cereals and crackers to some canned foods, contain refined sugar, white flour or cornflour in some form, hydrogenated fat and some salt.

Refined carbohydrates like cakes and biscuits are good examples of high-fat, high-sugar processed foods that are high in calories but low in nutritional value and should be avoided. Refined sugar is actively addictive and makes you crave an increased dose at ever-decreasing intervals. You are better off without it.

fat

Fat is complicated, but, to keep it simple, there are two kinds: good and bad. The good ones clean your arteries and help process the vitamins you ingest, as well as acting as a secondary energy source. The bad ones clog your arteries. All fats, good and bad, are high in calories, so even the good ones only need to be consumed in small amounts. Too much can be addictive. Too little makes your food unappetising and will lead to poor health.

Good fats are found in olive oil, flaxseed oil, fish oils, nuts, avocado and natural peanut butter. A few others you'll see advertised as high in omega 3 and omega 6. Your brain and body require a small daily dose of good fat.

A tablespoon of flaxseed oil per day and three meals with oily fish per week takes care of all your needs. Fat is very important but you don't need much of it.

Bad fats are, as a general rule, hard at room temperature and should be avoided. They include butter and cheese as well as the fat on meat. Eat them only in moderation and try skimmed milk or soy milk instead of full-fat. The archvillain among bad fats is hydrogenated fat. Nearly all processed food - pastries, pies, anything in batter, sauces and so on, and some vegetable oils - contain hydrogenated or 'trans fat', which in its basic form is margarine. This actively increases the plaque-producing LDL cholesterol that clogs arteries. Don't eat it. Shun solidified spreads or processed foods - especially things like pies or cheesecake.

To sum up:

- Eat food in its most natural, unprocessed state

- Eat five times a day – three main meals and two snacks

- Eat protein and carbohydrates at every meal

- Eat complex carbohydrates early in the day

- Eat fibrous carbohydrates (vegetables) later in the day

- Avoid sugar, processed food or hydrogenated fat

- Get your daily dose of good fat

- Keep your metabolic rate high by maintaining or building muscle

some good things to eat

porridge

In my opinion, this is the best breakfast you can have. It achieves a good balance of complex carbohydrates, protein and good fat. Cooked oats are a slow-release carbohydrate – exactly what you're looking for when you want to get in shape and stay that way. Porridge is delicious with fruit, cinnamon, crushed walnuts or even some flaxseeds, which will give your porridge a nice crunchy texture while adding those desirable 'good fats' we all need. If you tire of it, there are plenty of other whole-grain cereals out there. Look in a health-food store for barley, wheat, rye, oat bran and flax cereals (or a multigrain combination of these).

sweet potatoes

Full of flavour, natural, low in calories and packed with nutrients. These are a personal favourite of mine. Combine a sweet potato with a green vegetable and chicken breast for a perfect fat-burning, muscle-building meal.

potatoes

Potatoes are a complex carbohydrate, so they'll keep you going rather than giving you an energy surge. They contain vitamins and minerals and – especially if you leave the skins on – fibre. Boiled or baked, they're not high in calories. Eat a baked potato just as it is or with low-fat cottage cheese or any other healthy protein and a vegetable to make a complete meal.

rice

Brown rice is another great carbohydrate, so long as you avoid fried rice in favour of slow-cooked brown or basmati rice. A portion with vegetables and meat or fish will make a meal. Don't eat boil-in-the-bag rice or cheap white rice, which gives you a short burst of energy but leaves you wanting more. Also, remember to stick to the portion size and eat earlier in the day.

pasta

Whole-wheat pasta is better for you than white pasta; however, it is easy to eat too much of it – and it is calorie-dense. Pasta sauces add significantly to the calorie count too, so I would suggest that you limit pasta meals to two per week and keep to a sensible portion size (see the 1, 2, 3 method on page 53). Choose a tomato-based sauce as opposed to something like pesto.

If you have a lot of weight to lose – leave pasta out of your diet altogether.

100 per cent whole wheat and whole grain

You can eat small amounts of bread, as long as it's made of 100 per cent whole grain. The label must say '100% whole wheat' or '100% whole grain' as the first ingredient; it's full of nutrition and fibre.

Some people find that bread just doesn't agree with them. It can cause digestive difficulties and bloating. If you have this problem, or if you have a lot of weight to lose, you should leave bread out of your diet altogether.

green leafy vegetables

Fibrous carbohydrate – celery, broccoli, cabbage, lettuce, you name it – is the best carbohydrate to balance your diet with if you're on a fat-loss programme. It's virtually impossible to eat too many greens because they contain so few calories. So have plenty, mostly late in the day. If your last two meals of the day are steamed greens (or salad) and a lean protein like chicken, you'll find yourself losing fat quickly.

fresh fruit

Most of the carbs you eat should be complex or fibrous ones, but some simple carbohydrate such as whole fruit, which adds colour and variety, is fine even when you're on a fat-loss programme.

Although fruits release their energy quite quickly, they also have fibre and vitamins and most are low in calories compared to the complex carbs: an apple, peach, grapefruit or orange, for instance, will contain only 60 to 80 calories. The only exception is dried fruit. Things like raisins or dried figs are packed with concentrated sugar. It's unrefined sugar, and dried fruit is so fibrous that you're unlikely to consume lots of it, but even so eat it sparingly. Eat a protein such as cottage cheese with fresh fruit, to slow the energy release and make you feel full. An all-fruit (or mostly fruit) weight-loss programme won't work as well as one that emphasises green fibrous carbohydrates with lean protein; and like any 'diet' it will prove ultimately unsustainable, because it'll be boring and impractical.

skimmed milk and non-fat dairy

Whole-milk products are high in fat. If you want to maintain your weight stick to

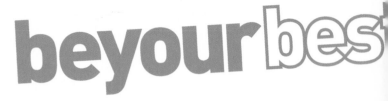

low-fat dairy produce. Even semi-skimmed milk still gets most of its calories from fat, but you could have non-fat cottage cheese as a protein instead of a serving of lean meat. Non-fat cheese can also boost the protein content of a meal. Yoghurt has less protein than cottage cheese, so a single serving of yoghurt would be a bit low in protein. However, yoghurt does have carbohydrate, and if mixed with some protein powder or cottage cheese will make a healthy and convenient snack.

egg whites and yolks

With zero fat, egg whites are as lean as lean proteins get, but whole eggs have a high fat and calorie content. All the fat is in the yolk, while the protein is split evenly between the yolk and the white.

One yolk for every three whites you eat is my guideline.

chicken and turkey breast

Chicken and turkey are the most popular protein sources among fat-loss seekers. Remove the skin and get the light meat found in the breasts. The thighs are higher in fat and calories. Your poultry should be grilled, roasted or microwaved rather than fried. That reconstituted chicken or turkey 'roll' you find in supermarkets is loaded with nutritionally valueless water, starch, hydrogenated fat, skimmed milk powder, preservatives and seasonings in order to add bulk and make it taste less revolting.

fish and seafood

Fish can provide the most valuable good fats of all and add variety to your diet. Eat it baked, grilled or poached. Most fish are very low in fat and high in protein. Some, such as salmon, mackerel, sardines, herring and trout, are high in beneficial oils and should be eaten two or three times a week. Shellfish such as prawn, crab, mussels and so on offer many of the same benefits and make a welcome change to egg white and chicken. When you're eating in restaurants, try ordering fish that isn't overwhelmed by a rich sauce or covered in batter.

spices and herbs, salt and dressings

Spices and herbs are delicious and of insignificant calorific value. Fresh parsley is particularly good for you and green herbs like coriander leaves add crunch. Fresh herbs are available almost anywhere, and, if you buy whole spices and grind them yourself, they keep longer.

Be wary of salt; you will find that most stock cubes and some 'seasonings' are largely salt. If you eat more than the recommended daily allowance of salt you risk raising your blood pressure (see Chapter 3), and too much doesn't do your kidneys any good, either. The more you avoid it, the less you'll find you want – it's addictive, like sugar, and will make you retain water.

Look for low-calorie versions of dressings, like balsamic vinegar, or mix your own - an oil and vinegar or oil and lemon dressing takes about ninety seconds to make and tastes better. If you are intolerant to lactose (milk sugar) check the labels of all sauces, because some do contain it. Or make your own sauce - it's quick and the result will keep for days in the fridge.

lean red meat

Choose only lean red meat, keep your portion sizes small, and it'll provide plenty of protein. But, if your main objective is fat loss, don't eat red meat more than once a week.

water

Drink lots - two or three glasses with every meal. When you're training drink water whenever you need it. Don't let yourself get thirsty.

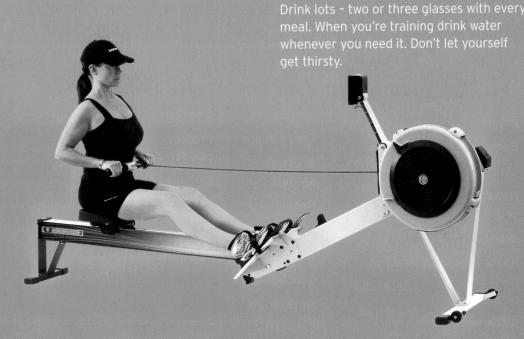

" Drink lots of water – two or three glasses with every meal. When you're training drink water whenever you need it. Don't let yourself get thirsty. "

good food choices at a glance

carbohydrates			protein	fat
starchy Slow release, high fibre, high nutrient	**fruit** Quick release, high nutrient, some fibre	**fibrous** High nutrient, low calorie		
Eat early in the day	Eat early in the day	Eat late in the day	Eat with all meals	Eat with two meals
Porridge	Apples	Asparagus	Fish	Flaxseed oil
Potatoes (white/red)	Blueberries	Broccoli	Egg whites	Fish fat (salmon, trout, herring or sardines)
Sweet potatoes	Strawberries	Okra	Chicken breast	
Beans	Bananas	Cauliflower	Shellfish	Olive oil
Lentils	Oranges	Green beans	Protein powder	Canola oil
Natural yoghurt	Raspberries	Brussels sprouts	Skimmed milk	Natural peanut butter
Brown rice	Nectarines	Peas	Low-fat cottage cheese	Nuts and seeds
100% whole-grain dry cereals	Plums	Cucumber		Avocado
100% whole-wheat or whole-grain pasta	Grapes	Squash		
100% whole-wheat bread and whole-grain products	Peaches	Cabbage		
	Cantaloupe	Mushrooms		
	Grapefruit	Courgette		
	Pears	Lettuce		
		Salads		
		Pepper, green or red		
		Tomatoes		
		Spinach		

what shouldn't i eat?

Anything that is:

● High calorie

● High fat

● High in refined sugar

● High in salt (sodium)

● Low in nutritional value

● High in flavour enhancers, artificial colours, improvers, flavouring or preservatives

Always read the label on the back – the small print. Junk foods have negative nutritional value. They subtract from the good you're doing when you pick the right foods. Anything high in refined sugar will spike your insulin levels. You'll have a quick boost followed by a slump in energy and a craving for more sugar. Don't even think of eating any of the following every day.

ice cream

Ice cream is loaded with bad fat, sugar and many more calories than you need, and most brands contain artificial additives. If you crave something sweet and frozen buy a fresh-fruit sorbet or sugar-free, low-fat frozen yoghurt.

fried foods

I don't mean a pan of heart-friendly garlic and onion sweated in olive oil as the basis of a healthy tomato soup. I mean fried, as in rashers of bacon and black pudding and a salty banger fried fast in half a pack of dodgy fat. This kind of sizzle destroys essential fatty acids. Also, margarine has replaced lard in the British frying pan and is even worse, because it is hydrogenated fat – vegetable oil, chemically treated to stay solid at room temperature – plus colour and flavour.

bacon and sausages

These are bad for your health. A rasher of bacon gives you 130 calories and 93% of them are saturated fat. As for 'reduced-fat bacon' – check the label. If the fat's reduced from 93 per cent to 50 per cent by some means, how terrific is that? Be suspicious. Stick with lean proteins.

hot dogs, fast food, burgers

Hot dogs (if you're lucky) are meat including fat, water, milk powder, sugar, salt and preservatives. Hamburgers are made from some of the fattiest meat available. If fast-food joints really served top-quality 'lean ground beef' as they often claim, they could call it steak tartare and charge five times the price. You can look for an alternative.

doughnuts, pastries and milk chocolate

If your goals are to reduce body fat and get healthier, these are not for you. Like ice cream, they contain an artery-clogging combination of refined sugar and saturated fats. The flour in doughnuts is white, the fat saturated, the sugar refined; pastries and chocolate are about the same.

white bread

Your body reacts to white bread as it does to refined sugar. Whole-grain breads (100 per cent wheat, rye, etc.) are another story. Anything made from cornflour or white or 'enriched' flour (many cereals and snack foods and crackers, as well as bread, pizza base, pies, thickened bottled sauces) will turn more quickly to fat than it would if it were made of whole-grain flour. If you're not sure whether a food is whole grain or not, simply read the ingredients list on the label. If the food really is whole grain, then the first ingredient will say something like '100% whole wheat'. To convert grains efficiently instead of putting on fat, give up white flour and insist on whole grain.

crisps, nachos and salty snacks

Your average crisp is potato starch and salt, with colorants and flavouring and the refined oil in which it is frazzled, but none of the nutritional value it would have were it a shaving of potato. These days you can find fat-free crisps at a health-food store, which are definitely an improvement. Put nachos and salted nuts on your 'Out' list too. Packaged and processed food is never as good as something you made yourself from healthy ingredients.

biscuits, cakes and pies

Biscuits, cakes and pies fall into the same categories as doughnuts – fat and sugar all in one neat little unhealthy package – no better than fried foods. Fat and sugar make the worst of all food combinations and they're both found in abundance in biscuits, cakes and pies. They also contain untold amounts of dangerous fatty acids. Save the cake for once a year on your birthday.

sugary breakfast cereals

A high percentage of breakfast cereals contain added sugar and some are more than 50 per cent sugar. Cereal manufacturers are clever in their marketing, and many cereals appear much healthier than they are when 'fortified' with vitamins and minerals. Leave them on the shelf. Look for 'no added sugar or salt' and learn to read the label.

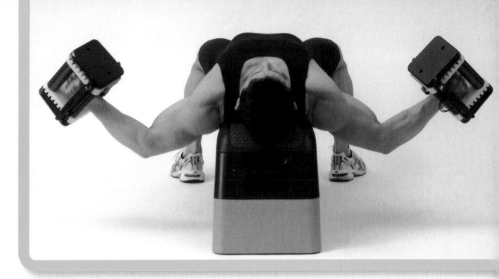

Remember: refined sugar contains neither vitamins, nor minerals, nor fibre. Just calories. It wreaks havoc with your blood-sugar levels; you risk mood swings. It increases your insulin level, which can also increase fat storage and prevent stored fat from being released. It is addictive; you find it hard to do without sweet things once you're used to them. You're likely to be buying cereals (or drinks; see below) for your children. Do you really want to get them addicted to sugar? Sugary foods cause hyperactivity, not to mention weight gain and tooth decay.

soft drinks

Soft drinks are mostly water, but the amount of sucrose and high fructose used to sweeten them is more than enough to do its share of damage. Liquid sugar piles on weight even faster than the granular kind. Several studies have shown that, when you consume liquid calories, you don't cut back on food. So the calories in soft drinks are not 'part of a balanced diet', but an addition to it. Liquid calories of all types are best avoided.

fruit drinks

It's label-reading time again. A fruit juice is what it says; a fruit drink is water and fruit juice with added sugar. And, when you see a fruit smoothie, read the ingredients. Some are exactly what they say: a blend of fresh fruit, freshly made. Others are fruit, plus sugar, preservative and colour.

It's easy to overconsume calories in fruit drinks, so I suggest you eat the fruit whole in its natural state and drink water.

alcohol

Alcohol contains almost twice the calories of carbohydrate, has no nutritional value and destroys your resolve. If you are trying to lose body fat, alcohol has no place in your diet. If you must have it, wait until you are in good shape, then save it for special occasions. Alcohol interferes with your sleep and significantly reduces the male hormone testosterone, leaving heavy drinkers with a beer belly and sometimes 'man breasts'.

bad food choices at a glance

bad carbohydrates	bad proteins	bad fats
Sweetened breakfast cereals with no whole grains	Hot dogs	Cream
	Salami	Sour cream
White bread or white bread products	Sausage	Cream cheese
	Bacon	Hard cheese
Crackers, muffins and baked goods made with white flour and hydrogenated oils	Luncheon meat	Palm oil
	Corned beef	Coconut oil
Desserts and puddings	Any processed meat	Palm kernel oil
Fizzy drinks made with sugar		Anything fried
		High-fat cuts of meat
Any sugar-sweetened drinks		Dairy products made from full fat
Alcoholic drinks		

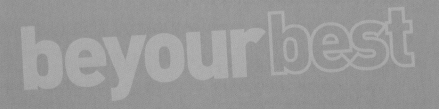

how much is too much?

Follow the 1, 2, 3 method of portion size for lunch and dinner. Imagine your plate is divided into four:

> 1 - protein fills the first quarter
>
> 2 - carbohydrate goes in the second
>
> 3 - a different carbohydrate goes in the third
>
> The fourth quarter should be empty. If it isn't, you're eating too much.
>
> The type of carbohydrate will differ depending on whether it's lunch or dinner.

Using my plan, you will eat three main meals - breakfast, lunch and dinner - with two snacks in-between. The structure of the meals may change during the specialisation phase (see step 4, page 114). For example, if you are trying to lose fat, you will be eating more fibrous and less starchy carbohydrates and, if you are trying to gain muscle, you may need to add an extra high-protein snack.

Eating right is about planning ahead so you have a healthy option rather than grabbing junk food for convenience. This can mean taking a lunchbox to work and occasionally using meal-replacement shakes. They are tasty, nutritious and convenient - and are a useful tool that will enable you to stay in control of your new eating regime.

some meal examples

My eating system is based on the following rules:

● **Breakfast:** choose a lean protein, plus a complex carbohydrate and a piece of fruit (optional)

● **Lunch:** choose a lean protein, plus a complex carbohydrate and a fibrous carbohydrate

● **Dinner:** choose a lean protein, plus a complex carbohydrate and a fibrous carbohydrate (or two fibrous carbohydrates if fat loss is the main goal)

● **Snacks:** refer to the list provided

Use the table on the following page as a template for structuring your meals, and remember to drink water with all meals.

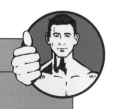

breakfasts

2 Weetabix with skimmed milk and a portion of fruit

Porridge (³/₄ cup) with skimmed milk (1 cup) and 1 piece of fruit

Scrambled eggs (1 yolk and 3 whites) on toast with tomatoes

Scrambled eggs (1 yolk with 3 whites) with baked beans (small tin)

Baked beans (small tin) on toast (1 slice)

Plain low-fat yoghurt (250g) with fruit

Poached eggs (1-2) on toast (eat only once per week)

Yoghurt (250g) with a scoop of your favourite flavour whey protein

Tea or coffee should be made with skimmed milk (or black) and no sugar (keep an eye on how many mugs you drink! - no more than 4 per day)

▟▟ Use the tables on these pages as inspiration for healthy meal ideas ▟▟

lunches and dinners

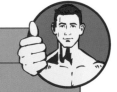

1 chicken breast with sweet potato (or rice) and salad

1 salmon fillet with baked potato (or rice) and broccoli

Cottage cheese (3 tablespoons/200g) with 1 sweet potato and chopped red onion

Tuna (1 tin) with tinned tomatoes (1 tin) and chopped mushrooms

Steak (lean) with spinach and boiled potatoes (or rice)

Omelette (1 yolk and 3 egg whites) with mushrooms and red peppers/onion

1 turkey breast with corn on the cob and swede/salad

On the basic plan you can eat starchy and fibrous carbohydrates with dinner, but when losing fat only eat starch up to lunchtime

snacks

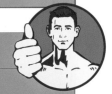

Fruit (1 piece) with nuts (a handful) – not dry roasted or salted!

Protein shake made with water or skimmed milk

Ryvita (x2) with cottage cheese (2 dessertspoons)

Rice cakes (x2) with natural peanut butter (1 level tablespoon)

Yoghurt (250g) with 1 scoop of flavoured protein powder/chopped nuts

Cottage cheese (2 dessertspoons) with baked beans/chopped fruit

Raw vegetables (no limit) with cottage cheese (100g)

Avoid 'health bars' – they generally contain too much sugar

an example of a healthy week

	Breakfast	Morning snack	Lunch	Afternoon snack	Dinner
monday	Weetabix with skimmed milk and fruit	Protein shake	Chicken with rice and spinach	Nuts and fruit	Tuna with tinned tomatoes and onion
tuesday	Scrambled eggs on toast with tomatoes	Yoghurt with chopped nuts	Cottage cheese with baked potato and salad	Protein shake	Mackerel with corn on the cob and broccoli
wednesday	Porridge with fruit and skimmed milk	Raw vegetables with cottage cheese	Chicken with boiled potatoes and carrots	Rice cake with natural peanut butter	Turkey with swede and spinach
thursday	Yoghurt with fruit and scrambled eggs	Ryvita with cottage cheese	Sweet potato with tuna and salad	Yoghurt with whey protein	Mushroom omelette and salad
friday	Baked beans on toast	Yoghurt with fruit	Chicken with boiled potatoes and peas	Ryvita with cottage cheese	Steak with green beans and spinach
saturday	Yoghurt with whey protein	Rice cake with natural peanut butter	Tuna with brown rice and asparagus	Yoghurt with chopped nuts	Cottage cheese with red onion and corn on the cob
sunday	Poached eggs on toast	Fruit and nuts	Salmon with sweet potato and salad	Protein shake	Chicken with cabbage and marrow

Of course, you can eat the same meals every day if you have a particular favourite and use dressings such as flaxseed or olive oil on your salads and vegetables.

shopping

I've heard people say they can't resist sneaking off to the biscuit tin. I admit, it takes a class-A brain to devise a solution to this problem. Personally, I do not have a biscuit tin and don't buy biscuits. It seems to work. And do not use your children as an excuse. Having kids is even more reason to not have a biscuit tin. They look to you for guidance. Do them a favour and do not lead them into habits that, long term, may lead to obesity, type-2 diabetes and all the other avoidable illnesses that are created through long-term junk-food habits. If you shop for food when you are hungry, the store has a built-in advantage. Eat first, take your time, consider the nutritional value of what you're buying and read the ingredients. To help with your shopping, make reference to the following chart for some healthy alternative options.

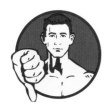 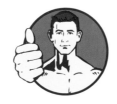

poor choice	choose instead
Whole milk	Skimmed milk
Ice cream	Low-fat, non-fat or sugar-free frozen yoghurt, or fruit sorbet
Whole eggs	Egg whites or one yolk to every three whites
Cheese	Low-fat cottage cheese
Tuna in oil	Tuna packed in water
Fried chicken	Skinless chicken breast
Rump steak	Fillet steak (no more than once per week)
Bacon, sausage, hot dogs	Cold cuts of turkey and chicken breast

poor choice	choose instead
Buttered popcorn	Light microwaved or air-popped popcorn
Cream crackers	100% whole-wheat or rye bread
Doughnuts	Whole-wheat Ryvita, rice cakes
Fruit drinks	100% fruit juice/water
Fizzy drinks	Diet fizzy drinks (both are best avoided)
Canned fruit in syrup	Fresh fruits
Table sugar	Sweet N Low or honey
Flavoured, sweetened porridge	Old-fashioned whole oats (Quaker Oats)
Sugary cereals	Shredded Wheat, or any whole-grain, low-sugar cereal
Supermarket oils	Extra-virgin olive oil or flaxseed oil
Mayonnaise	Low- or non-fat mayonnaise
Chips	Baked or boiled potatoes

eating out

There's no need to avoid eating at restaurants just because you're eating smart.

You can construct meals of lean proteins and healthy carbohydrates just as easily at a restaurant as you can in your own kitchen. You just need to know what to ask for. Read menus, watch for sneaky fat, know how your food is prepared and don't hesitate to explain exactly what you want and how you want it prepared. Pay attention to the amount they're giving you. In some restaurants your plate will arrive spilling over, and in others you'll be presented with two olives and a single unlovely mushroom on a minuscule 'bed of wilted spinach', pursued by a big bill. Neither extreme is good, but, if you think you may get too much, ask for your main course to be the size of a starter. And when you definitely don't want extra calories from unseen butter and oil used in cooking, check that you can get what you want. These days most restaurants have plenty of healthy options within their normal menu. Some fast-food restaurants now have salad bars, low-calorie dressings, grilled sandwiches and sugar-free frozen yoghurt.

Use the Dos & Don'ts chart to help you eat healthier when dining out.

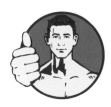

do

- Order food described as grilled, poached, roasted, baked or steamed

- Order whole-grain breads

- Order your vegetables steamed

- Order fresh fruit (no whipped creams or toppings)

- Order grilled (not fried) chicken breasts and make sure the skin is removed

- Order red pasta sauces instead of creamy white sauces

- Order starters containing chicken, fish, seafood, rice, potatoes and vegetables

- Order your baked potatoes with no butter, no sour cream and no bacon bits

- Order green and tossed salads without the high-fat toppings (bacon bits, cheese, croutons)

- Order low-calorie salad dressings

- Order beverages such as low-fat skimmed milk, diet drinks, water, tea and coffee

- Eat small portions (stick to the 1,2,3 method)

- Use freely spices, pepper, herbs, mustard, lemon juice and vinegar

- Order desserts including frozen yoghurt, sorbet and fresh fruit

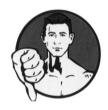

don't

- Order restaurant or fast-food burgers – they are usually loaded with fat and are very high in calories (instead choose a grilled chicken or turkey breast sandwich and to improve further throw away half the bun, or better still throw it all away and add a salad)

- Order cheese- or cream-based soups (instead choose clear, broth-based soups)

- Order foods described as buttered, buttery, in butter sauce, fried, batter-dipped or in its own gravy

- Order rich, creamy sauces

- Put croutons, bacon bits, ham, creamy dressing and other high-fat toppings on salads

- Order croissants, pastries, biscuits or buttered rolls

- Order traditional desserts (if you must, split one dessert with a friend)

- Feel that you must eat everything on your plate

beyourbest

❝❝You can construct meals of lean proteins and healthy carbohydrates just as easily at a restaurant as you can in your own kitchen❞❞

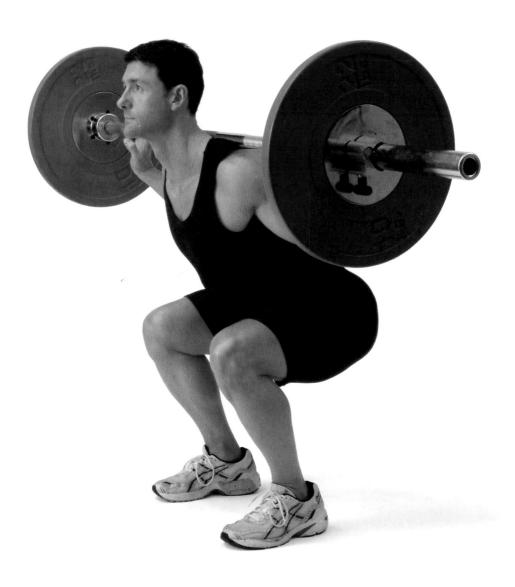

to be your best

- Eat food in its most natural, unprocessed state

- Eat five times a day (three meals and two snacks)

- Eat protein and carbohydrates at every meal

- Eat complex carbohydrates early in the day

- Eat fibrous carbohydrates later in the day

- Avoid eating sugar, processed food or hydrogenated fat

- Don't overeat (remember the 1, 2, 3 method)

- Get your daily dose of good fat

- Keep your metabolic rate high by maintaining or building muscle

- Drink two cups of water with every meal (and don't exceed four cups of tea or coffee per day)

Remember that you are in charge: not the supermarket, not the advertiser, not the restaurateur, but you – it's your money, your body and your life. Combining carbohydrates and protein not only ensures that you are getting the nutrients you need, but it also slows the release of carbohydrates. This maintains energy levels and controls appetite at the same time. Eating unprocessed food keeps your metabolic rate high because your body uses energy in the digestive process.

Don't diet. Just eat smart.

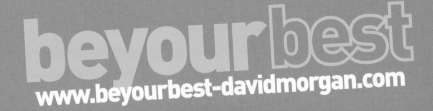

5

types of training

> **There are two types of training you need to use if you are going to be your best. They are CV (cardiovascular) and resistance/strength training.**

beyourbest

cardiovascular

Cardiovascular or CV training is also referred to as aerobic, which means with oxygen.

For the purpose of this book CV relates to steady rhythmical movements that elevate the heart rate for between ten and twenty minutes. This can be achieved with or without special equipment. However, I particularly favour the stationary bike and indoor rowing machine.

I like these because they are measurable in terms of resistance, they're weatherproof and non-ballistic (kind to your joints).

Some of you will want to run, and that's OK providing you are not overweight and do not have any joint problems. Having said that, I still think that the stationary bike or indoor rowing are the safest and best options. If you are overweight,

cycling and rowing are the only options! I am promoting getting in great shape, staying in shape and being your best for life, not wearing out your joints or injuring yourself.

> **Note** - If you have been running all your life and have not experienced any problems, that's fine. However, do not be closed off to the idea of including some cycling or rowing. The different type of training is good for the mind and body. If you have stagnated with your running, are bored or have some niggling pains, then a change for a couple of months to bike or rower may be just what you need to get rid of the niggles and break the plateau.

what rate should you work at?

You should work at a rate that gets you slightly out of breath, but allows you to just about hold a conversation. Or you can use your pulse as a guide. To calculate this, subtract your age from 220 – this will give you your maximum heart rate.

You should work at 65 to 85 per cent of that maximum, depending on your level of fitness. If you are 40 years of age, the calculation would be as follows:

> **220 - 40 = 180, your maximum heart rate**
>
> **180 x 0.65 = 117, your lower exercising heart rate**
>
> **180 x 0.85 = 153, your higher exercising heart rate**

If you are new to exercise, work nearer your lower range, and, as you get fitter and more experienced, you can work near the higher range.

You should note that this calculation is just a guide. Some of you will be able to work very comfortably in a higher range.

when should you do it and how often?

Your chance of success is much greater if you schedule a time that cannot be affected by other things in your life. From my experience, morning before work or evening immediately after work – i.e. before you go home to distractions – are the best times to do your exercise.

Morning is good because it will kick-start your day. There is also a theory that you will burn more calories at this time of the day, which may or may not be true. But, most important, if you do it in the morning it's done and nothing can get in the way later in the day. You think you don't have time – GET UP EARLIER!

CV training is very useful for increasing heart and lung fitness. It's also great for burning excess calories when trying to lose body fat or maintain a healthy weight. Combined with weight training and smart eating, it is an important component to being your best.

The Rotational and Progressive system (see Chapter 9) builds CV into your workout.

resistance/strength training

"Muscle gain plus smart eating is the key to long-term fat loss, and maintaining muscle is one of the major factors in staying young."

Resistance training involves using free weights, machines or your bodyweight for resistance and is classed as anaerobic, or without oxygen.

It is useful for increasing and/or maintaining strength and muscle mass. It has also been proven over time to increase bone density and tendon and ligament strength.

This is the type of exercise that defines your body. Muscle and fat gives our body its shape. Therefore, to get the best shape, we need to build muscle and lose fat. The most effective way of doing this is to combine weight training with aerobic work and smart eating.

Something else you should consider is that bodies with more muscle have higher metabolic rates. This means that people with more muscle burn more calories, not only in the gym, but also at rest.

We have already covered this but it is a key point so I am going to go over it once more. Muscle is living tissue. Living tissue needs fuel and, therefore, the more you have, the more fuel you will burn. Also, the more muscle you have and the fitter you are, the harder you will be able to work during your training sessions and the more calories you will burn.

Let's quantify this so it makes more sense.

For every extra pound of muscle you have you will burn about an extra 50 calories per day. That's an extra 50 calories just for it being there. So, if you gain 7 pounds of muscle you will burn 350 extra calories per day without doing anything. This is another long-term benefit of weight training and illustrates what a powerful weight-controlling mechanism extra muscle mass is.

It has been said that the average person over the age of thirty loses about 10 per cent of their muscle mass per decade. Weight training stops and reverses this process. Loss of muscle mass is the main reason that people struggle with their weight in later life.

Small changes make a huge difference over time. People do not get fat overnight. Getting very fat is caused by eating a little bit too much over a long period of time, with a small drop in activity levels and a loss of muscle mass as you get older.

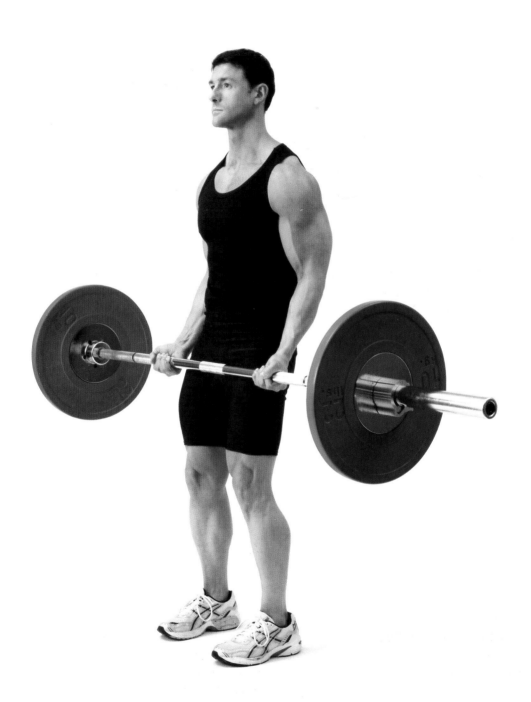

very small shift in your daily habits. Weight training is the most effective long-term way to lose fat and keep it off for life.

being your best

In practice, to be in your best shape ever you need to combine smart eating with CV and resistance/strength training. That's the secret formula used by fitness models, bodybuilders, top athletes and anyone who wants to stay in great shape.

Training systems, repetitions and sets, correct exercise, form, rest and diet are all very important and if you get them wrong you will not make the progress you desire. However, you also need a specific training strategy that allows you to continue to progress steadily until you reach your goal. If you just keep adding weight, doing the same repetitions and the same exercises you will very quickly hit a brick wall in terms of progress. The aim of the Rotational and Progressive system is to show you how to structure your training so this does not happen for a very long time (obviously there are limits, but very few of us will ever reach them, or want to).

The Rotational and Progressive method involves the rotation of exercises, repetitions, rest periods and eating habits to maintain progress – it is necessary to change from time to time. If you stay on the same regime for too long, your gains will dry up, you will get bored and you may even start to get little niggly overuse aches and pains.

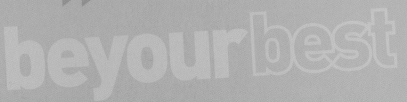

For every extra pound of muscle you have you will burn about an extra 50 calories per day. That's an extra 50 calories just for it being there

beyourbest

6

motivation and goal setting

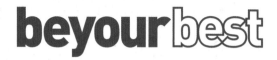

beyourbest

> ## "A great pleasure in life is doing what people say you cannot do"
>
> ## Walter Bagshot (1826–1877)

You have the ability to achieve almost anything you like, providing you have sustained motivation on your side.

what if i don't feel like doing it?

If you want something badly enough you will do it even when you do not feel like it. I think that accepting there will be days that you will not feel like training is realistic. But the people in life that succeed will acknowledge this fact, but do it anyway.

People get bored with exercise because they have unreasonable expectations. They want results too quickly and get disappointed when it takes longer. If you work to a plan you will see progress, first in terms of increased levels of fitness, and then changes in your body shape. Providing you can see your progress, you will keep training.

The Rotational and Progressive system gives you that plan.

It is important to know what you want. If you keep your eye on the goal and see yourself slowly moving towards it you will stay motivated. You also need to know what you do not want – i.e. a fat, unhealthy body that will eventually affect your quality of life or, even worse, end it prematurely.

staying motivated

Most people fail to reach their goal because it does not fit their time frame, or because the effort required is too much. Be ambitious but also be realistic.

Motivation is a strange subject. What motivates us? Why do some people succeed in their lives while others fail?

These are tough questions, with more than one answer. Over the last fifteen years of personal training I have found the two biggest motivators to be vanity and fear of premature death. I have also discovered that most people wait for a problem to happen before doing anything about it. Let me explain. Most people only get motivated when they have had the heart attack or had their partners walk out! Very few people train just to stop those things from happening in the first place.

Even top athletes find it hard to motivate themselves sometimes. When I was training for the Olympic and Commonwealth Games I never missed a training session unless I was genuinely ill. That doesn't mean I always felt like training. In fact, there were many times I wanted to skip a session. So why didn't I? Well, it was because, although I didn't like losing (who does?), I hated the thought of losing and knowing that I hadn't done my best in terms of contest preparation.

Whatever you do, you have to be doing for you

The trick is to have a definite goal and a plan that will support you in achieving that goal. Then stick to the plan on the understanding that at some point you will not want to do it. Not wanting to train some days is inevitable; you must now decide that when this happens (and believe me, it will) you are going to do it anyway.

Human beings are creatures of habit. Our habits can make or break us. They can support us in the achievement of our goals, or they can destroy us. Success is all about developing the right habits and sticking to them.

There is no doubt that changing habits can be very difficult. We all know that smoking is bad for us yet many people continue to smoke and many kids continue to take up the habit. The same is true of having a sedentary lifestyle and a diet of fast food. On an intellectual level we all know these things are harming us, yet many of us continue the behaviour.

So how can we change our bad habits? Perhaps the first step is to actually acknowledge them and what they are doing to us, and then ask ourselves if that's what we want long term. If it is, then fine, but if not you will have to make a conscious effort to replace your old destructive habits with new ones that will support you in your future goals and help you to be your best.

This involves conquering your most difficult opponent – YOU!

goal setting and designing your plan

Goal setting and plan design are important parts of staying motivated. Allowing yourself to acknowledge successful steps on the way to achieving your ultimate goal is a very strong motivational tool. Setting your goals and planning your eating and training are very important. In fact, if you do not set your goals and design your plan you will fail.

Your goal should be to eat smart and to train. This book does the planning side of the training regimes for you. Follow this, get fit – and stay motivated.

'If you fail to plan you plan to fail'

Keep a record of everything you do in your workouts. You can also keep a food diary until you get used to smart eating.

Chapter 9 includes training and diet regimes to suit all goals. It also takes you through a 4-step process. Steps 1 to 3 last for 8 weeks each, so will take 24 weeks to complete. Everyone should go through this initial 24 weeks. At the end of the 24 weeks you will have learned the exercises, increased your strength and got into the habit of smart eating. This is your foundation. It will be time to redo all your measurements and photos. Look back on your training and eating plan and ask yourself if you are happy with the results and if you have followed the plan.

This is important. Make sure you are honest with yourself when asking yourself: 'Did I follow the plan properly?' Remember this includes eating and training.

If the answer is no, list all the areas you feel that you fell down on and ask yourself why. Then determine what you can do now to enable yourself to excel in those areas.

Now list all the areas that you made progress in:

- Increased strength (be specific, e.g. 10kg (22lb) on your bench press)

- Increased aerobic ability (be specific, e.g. lower pulse rate and higher work rate)

- Measurements (e.g. reduced waist, increased chest)

- Bodyweight or, more importantly, body-fat levels (use the W2W chart in Chapter 2)

It's very important that you list these things so you know what you have achieved, and you know which areas to work on during step 4 of the Rotational and Progressive System – Specialisation (see page 114).

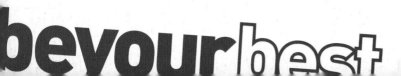
beyourbest

It is at this point that you assess where you want to go. I believe you have three choices:

1. **You will be happy with where you are now and just want to stay there**

2. **You will want to gain more muscle**

3. **You will want to lose more fat**

Step 4 will show how to achieve your ultimate goal once you have reassessed where you are and where you want to be.

This is an important process and, if done properly, will enable you to develop a tremendous self belief in your ability. Your feelings of achievement and the fact that you are in control of your health and fitness will be a great motivation.

one final thing for you to think about . . .

Many of you will be happy to just maintain a good level of fitness. Be careful, though, how you measure your progress. I had a client who had been with me for several years. He felt that the fact he was doing 'the same' things at the age of fifty as he was when he was forty was a negative thing.

I explained that actually this should be considered a huge achievement, as most people's ability to train deteriorates significantly as they get older.

You won't achieve PBs every training session, and some days will be hard work. There will be times when you do not feel like training and times when you will not eat perfectly. Do not beat yourself up about this because we become what we do for most of the time. For example, eating one healthy meal a month and training once every two months will not make you fit and healthy, in the same way that missing the odd session and eating the occasional junk food will not have a major impact.

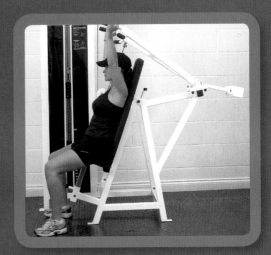

"Many of you will be happy to just maintain a good level of fitness. Be careful, though, how you measure your progress"

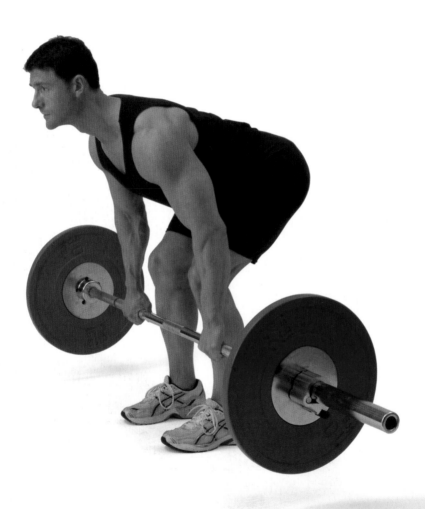

7

the exercises and how to perform them

beyourbest

When using weights you should take two seconds on the upwards movement and two seconds to lower the weights. You should exhale during the effort part of the exercise, i.e. as you lift the weight, breathe out, and breathe in as you lower the weight. The exception to this rule is the squat. During this exercise, take a deep breath before bending the legs to 90 degrees and hold it until you start the upwards drive. The reason for this is to keep the chest up and the body rigid during the exercise.

shoulders exercises
seated barbell press

Sit on the bench with your feet flat on the floor. Hold the barbell with a slightly wider than shoulder-width grip at shoulder height, elbows out and palms facing forward. Press the barbell to straight arms, and then lower slowly to the starting position.

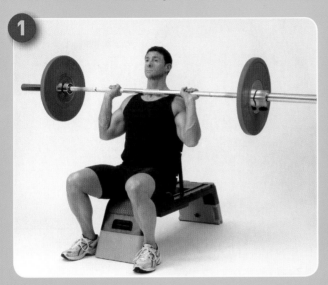

TIP
Keep the movement strict. Do not arch your back when pressing the barbell over your head.

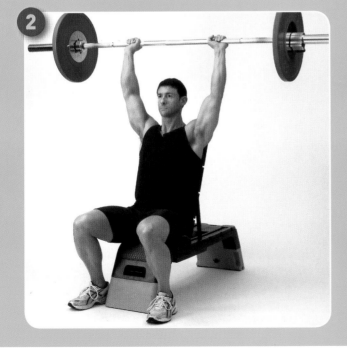

seated dumbbell press

Sit on the end of the bench with your feet flat on the floor. Hold a dumbbell in each hand, at shoulder height, elbows out, and palms facing forward. Press the dumbbells up and in, so they nearly touch above your head. Don't let the weights stray back and forth. Press the weights up until your arms are almost straight. Then, slowly lower the dumbbells to the starting position.

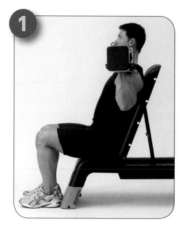

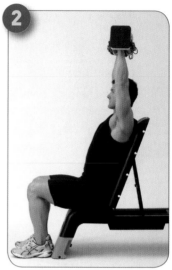

TIP
Dumbbells may feel hard to control to begin with. As you develop your stabilising muscles it will become easier and you will gain complete control.

barbell upright row

Stand holding barbell with an overhand grip, shoulder-width apart. Lift straight up, keeping it close to your body, until the bar reaches your chest. Lower under control to starting position.

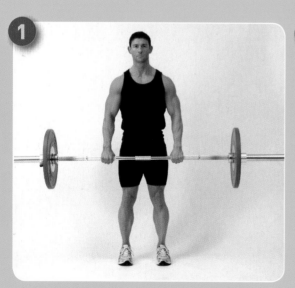

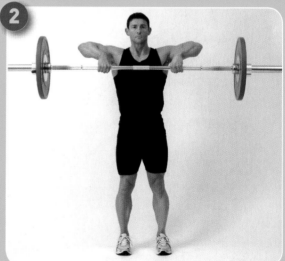

TIP
Remember to keep your back straight throughout this exercise and do not swing the body.

machine press

Adjust the seat so that the handrails are at shoulder height. Grab the handrails and push up to almost full extension. Return to the starting position.

TIP
Keep the muscles under tension all the time by not quite lowering the weight stack fully.

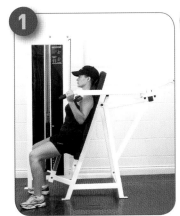

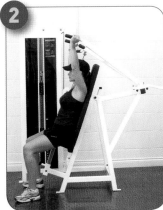

TIP
Do not expect to lift huge weights in this exercise because you are isolating the deltoid muscle. It's harder than you'd expect!

dumbbell side raises

Hold the dumbbells at your side while standing in an upright position. Raise the dumbbells out to the side to shoulder height, keeping your arms straight throughout the whole movement. Pause for a count of one, then lower.

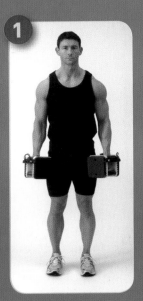

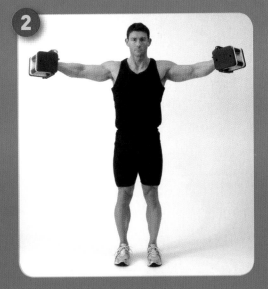

barbell dead lift

Stand over the barbell, feet hip-width apart, with the bar just touching your shin. Bend your knees, lean forward, and grasp the bar with a shoulder-width grip.

With a straight and flat back, keep the body tight and begin the lift by driving with the legs. Straighten up until you are standing upright, with your chest out and shoulders back. To lower the weight, bend the knees, lean forwards from the waist and touch the weight to the floor before beginning the next lift.

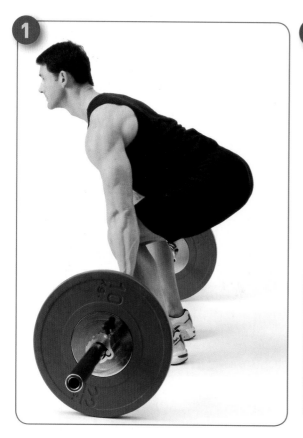

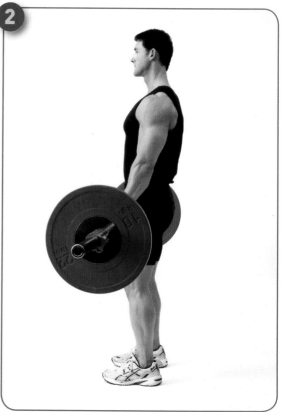

TIP
Keep your head up with your eyes looking forwards throughout the movement and keep your back flat.

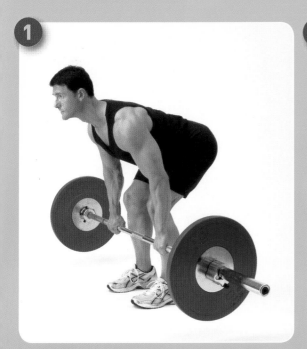

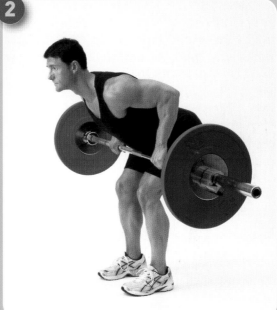

barbell bent over rows

Hold the bar with an overhand grip with your feet shoulder-width apart. Keep your back flat and unlock your knees. Now bend forwards at the hips keeping your back flat until your back is 45 degrees to the floor. Pull the barbell to your waist and then lower to the starting position under control.

TIP
Keep your head up and your body rigid at all times.

www.beyourbest-davidmorgan.com
beyourbest

dumbbell bent over rows

Start with your right foot flat on the floor and your left knee resting on a flat bench. Then lean forwards so you're supporting the weight of your upper body with your left arm on the bench. Reach down and pick up a dumbbell with your right hand. Look straight ahead in order to keep your back straight. Concentrate on pulling your elbow as far back as it can go. The dumbbell should end up roughly parallel with your torso. After you have 'rowed' the dumbbell up as far as you can, slowly lower it to the starting position. After you complete the planned number of reps for your right arm, follow the same instructions for your left.

TIP
Your back should be almost parallel with the floor during this exercise.

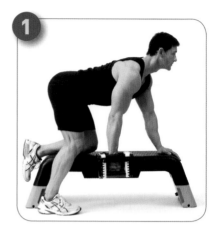

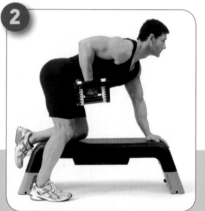

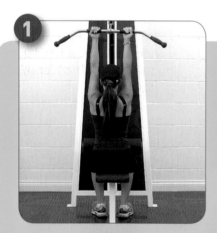

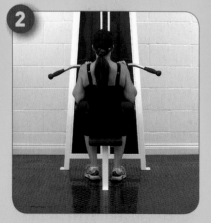

lat pull downs

Seated on a pull-down machine, reach up and take a shoulder-width grip with your palms facing you. From this stretched position, pull the bar down to your upper chest while contracting your back muscles and keeping your elbows in close to your body. Then let the weight back up, resisting it as you straighten your arms. As you finish the rep, your arms should be fully extended, and your lats will be stretched.

TIP
Lean back slightly as you pull down, keeping your chest high, and your abs and lower back tight.

chest exercises
barbell bench press

Lie down on a bench, and firmly position your feet flat on the floor a little wider than shoulder-width. You may wish to position your feet on the bench to stop your back from arching.

Using a grip broader than shoulder-width, hold the barbell, with your elbows locked out, right over the middle of your chest. Start by lowering the weight slowly to a point in the middle of your chest (aim for your nipples). Control the weight as you lower it, make contact with the mid-chest area and immediately drive the weight back up.

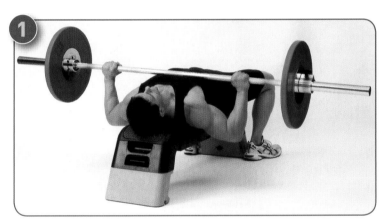

TIP
Don't bounce the barbell off your chest – stay in control of the entire movement. **Important – you must use a 'spotter' (training partner) for this exercise.**

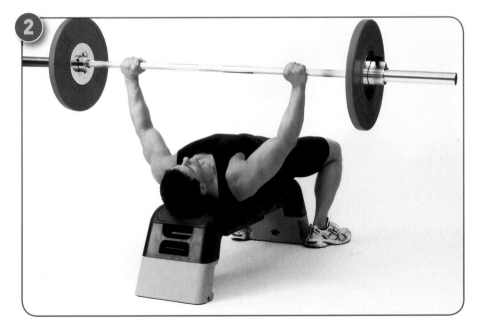

barbell incline bench press

Lean back, and get firmly situated on an incline bench. Lower the barbell to your mid-chest under control, and then drive up to the starting position.

TIP
Because of the angle and the leverage, you won't be able to lift as much as you can on the flat barbell bench press. **You will need a 'spotter' for this exercise.**

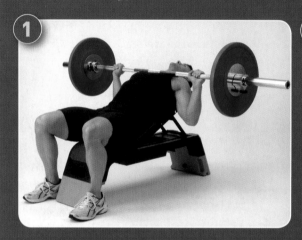

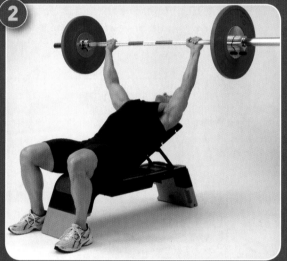

dumbbell bench press

Lie on your back on a bench, holding a dumbbell in each hand. Bring the weights to a point just above your shoulders, palms facing towards your feet and elbows out. Press the weights straight up until they're locked out right over your mid-chest (not over your face and not over your stomach). Then slowly lower them until your elbows drop below the level of the bench.

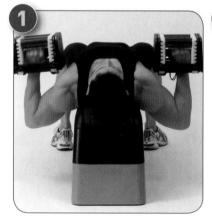

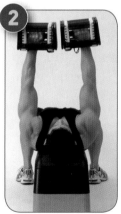

TIP
If you are training on your own, use this exercise instead of the barbell bench press – you can't get trapped underneath dumbbells.

machine bench press

Sit comfortably in the chair. Grip the handlebars, with your elbows at shoulder height.

Push the handlebars away until your arms are fully extended. Return the handlebars to your starting position.

TIP
If the machine has a foot pedal or bar, depress it to bring the handlebars into position and keep your head on the seat.

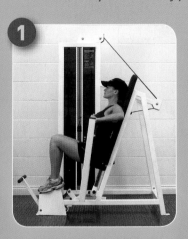

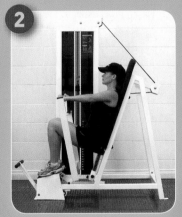

dumbbell flys

Lie flat on the bench with the dumbbells in the position shown, knuckles facing out. Slightly unlock the arms and lower arms into position 2, until you feel a stretch. Drive the arms back to position 1 under control.

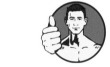

TIP
Lower the dumbbells slowly into position 2 – so you don't overstretch and pull a muscle.

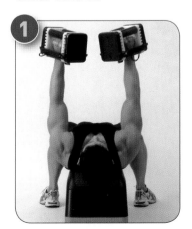

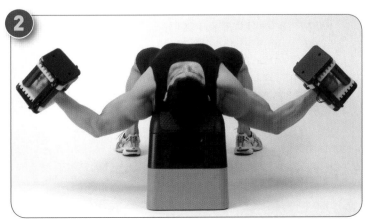

abdominal exercises
crunch

Start by lying on your back with your knees bent and feet resting flat on the floor. Gently position your hands behind your head to support it, not to pull on it. Don't lock your hands behind your head! Focus your mind on contracting the abdominal muscles before you even begin to lift your shoulders up off the floor. Contracting the abdominal muscles, curl the shoulders up and forward, until the upper back starts to lift off the floor. Concentrate on flexing the abdominal muscles when you are lifting the shoulders up, imagining you're trying to make a dent in the floor with your lower back, and let that contraction pull your shoulders off the ground. Hold the contracted position for a second before slowly returning to the starting position.

reverse crunch

Begin by lying on your back, knees bent and feet together, about six inches above the floor. Put your hands by your side flat on the floor with your palms facing down. Keeping your feet close to your hips, contract your abs while you slowly curl your lower body up towards your shoulders, gradually rolling your hips off the floor. Exhale when you contract the abs, so your rib cage will drop and allow for a more intense muscle contraction. Keep flexing the abs until your hips and lower back are just slightly off the floor. Hold that position for a count of one, and flex as hard as you can! Then slowly lower your hips back to the starting position, take a breath and repeat. The slower you do this exercise, the better it works.

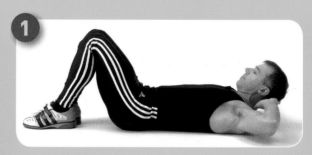

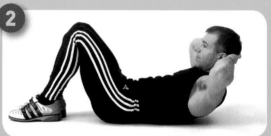

TIP
Do not try to sit all the way up. You can increase the difficulty of this exercise by holding a weight behind your head.

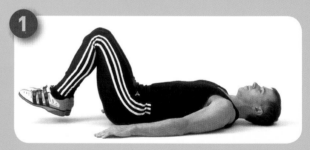

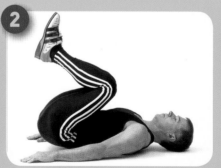

TIP
You can increase the difficulty of the reverse crunch by holding a small dumbbell between your feet or lying on an incline bench.

machine crunch

Adjust the height of the seat to suit your proportions (the pivot point of the upper part of the machine should be about shoulder height).

Sit on the machine, hook your feet behind the crosspieces or keep them flat on the floor (depending on the machine) and take hold of the handles. Curl your upper body downwards, flexing the abs. Hold this position for a count of one, then slowly release, lowering the weight stack under control back to the starting position.

TIP
Make sure you complete the full range of movement for this to be completely effective, and increase the weight when you reach the required rep range.

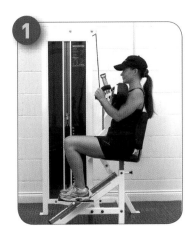
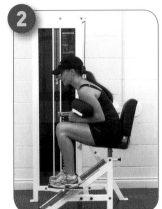

arm exercises

I have only included three specific arm exercises, two for the biceps and one for the triceps, because the arms are involved in all of the shoulder and chest and some of the back exercises.

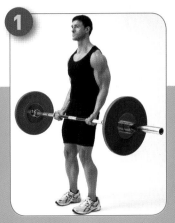

barbell curl

Stand with your feet shoulder-width apart, and hold the bar with an underhand grip. Curl the bar towards your shoulders and then lower under control.

TIP
Do not swing your body and keep your upper arms close into your sides at all times.

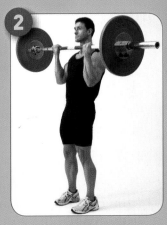

seated dumbbell curl

Sit on the edge of a bench with your arms at your sides, a dumbbell in each hand. With your palms facing upwards, curl your arms, lifting the dumbbells towards your shoulders. Let your biceps do the work. Then lower the dumbbells slowly to the starting point.

TIP
During the curl, keep your upper arms and torso still – there will be some movement, but avoid swinging the weight up (a common mistake).

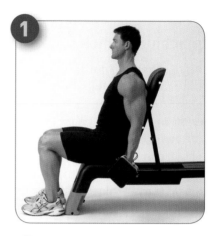

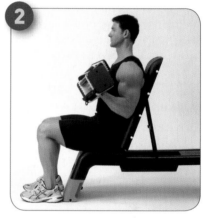

dumbbell lying triceps press

To begin, lie down on a flat bench with a dumbbell in each hand, positioned over your forehead. Next, lower the dumbbells either side of your head. It's important you go slow on this exercise and pause for a count of one, in both the fully stretched and contracted positions.

TIP
Performed properly, this is one of the best triceps exercises you can do.

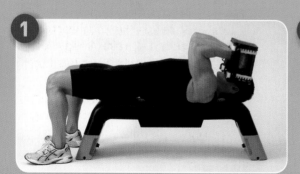

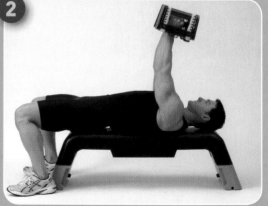

leg exercises

barbell squat

Position your feet slightly wider than shoulder-width apart. Rest the barbell on the back of your shoulders, not on your neck, and hold it in position in your hands. Keeping your chin up, eyes looking forwards and back straight, take a deep breath and hold it while bending your knees. Lower your hips until your thighs are parallel with the floor, pause and lift the weight back up, breathing out as you stand.

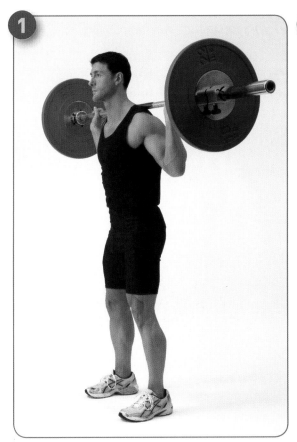

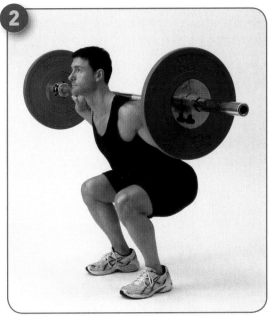

TIP
To get the best leg workout on this exercise, keep your back straight, your head up and your chest high – do not lean over. Please note, this is a very effective and demanding exercise. Do not be surprised if your legs are sore after the first few sessions of squat.

dumbbell squat

Hold two dumbbells at your sides, with your palms facing in. Stand with your feet about shoulder-width apart. While keeping your shoulders, back and head upright, bend your legs at the knees and lower your hips until your thighs are parallel with the floor. Then, pushing from your heels, lift yourself back up to the starting position. Keep your back as straight as possible throughout this exercise.

TIP
Use a bench to gauge how far to go with the squat. You should not sit down – just touch lightly before standing again.

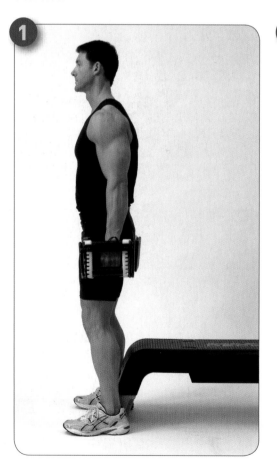

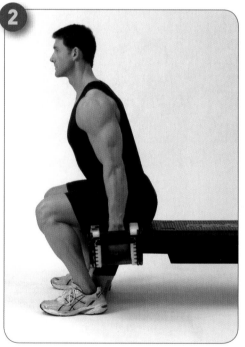

leg press

Position yourself on the seat of a leg-press machine, placing your feet about shoulder-width apart, toes slightly pointed out on the pressing platform. Slowly lower the weight to a point where you are comfortable. Then press the weight back to the starting position. This is a great leg exercise.

TIP
Be sure to push from your heels, not your toes, and don't quite lock your knees at the top – this keeps the muscles tense at all times.

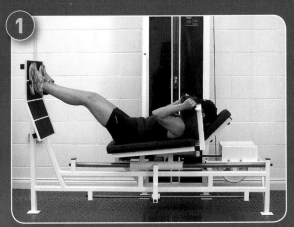

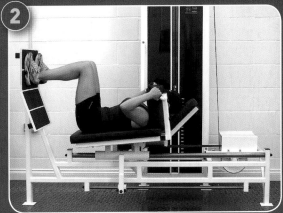

dumbbell calf raises

Position yourself in front of something that you can hold on to for stability, e.g. a wall or an incline bench. Hold a dumbbell in one hand and stand on one leg. Raise yourself up on to your toes, hold for a count of one and then lower.

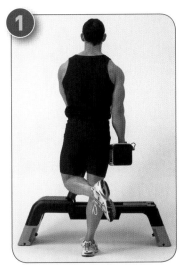

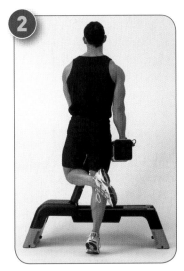

TIP
For a wider range of movement, stand with your toes on a four-inch wooden block. You can start off using both legs and then progress to doing them single-legged, and finally single-legged with a dumbbell.

cardiovascular exercise

rowing

On the first part of the drive, keep the body tight, your head fixed and your arms straight (see pictures 1 to 3). On the recovery, straighten your arms before you bend your knees (picture 6).

TIP
Remember, the recovery is just setting you up for the next drive. It may help initially to think the following when learning to row: 1 to 2 are recovery and 3 is the drive. Do not rush 1 or 2.

1. **Straighten arms**

2. **Move body forwards**

3. **Drive with the legs on straight arms**

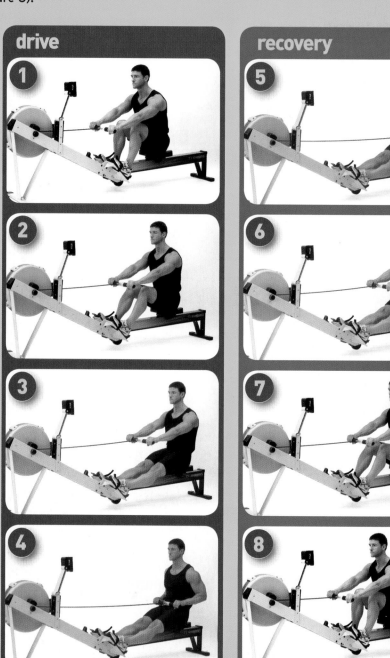

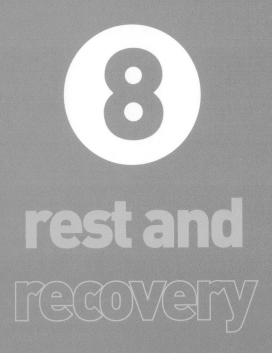

8

rest and
recovery

> **'Without enough rest and recovery your training is a waste of time'**
>
> **Exercise is the stimulus; however, rest is when the body adaptation actually takes place. Rest is when your muscle grows and your strength increases. I cannot stress enough how important it is to get adequate rest for recovery.**

If you do not get enough rest, at best your progress will stop. At worst you will get run down, ill, injured or all three.

There are several things that will tell you when you are not getting enough recovery time:

● Elevated pulse in the morning

● General tiredness

● Sore throat

● Your legs will feel heavy

● You may experience a lack of enthusiasm

● Your progress will come to a standstill or you may even see a regression in results

Take your pulse every morning as soon as you wake up. If it is six beats or more per minute higher than normal, you could be overtraining or have a low-level infection. This is a sign to slow down.

If you experience overtraining you should take one week off. During this week concentrate on eating well and getting more sleep. Then reassess your training routine and decide what needs to change so you can avoid further bouts of overtraining. There are several strategies you could use:

Take an extra day's rest between sessions – It may be that simple. For progress to continue you just require another 24 hours to recuperate. In some cases you may need to take more than an extra day, especially if you are training at a very high level. This is because the fitter and stronger you are, the harder you will be able to work in your sessions. This extra hard work will need more recovery time. Although we can increase our levels of

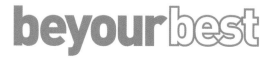

fitness significantly, we are limited when it comes to improving recovery times, especially as we get older. It seems to go against logic, but less really can be more.

Change your exercises – You may just have got used to the exercises and need a change. Usually after about eight weeks you will need to change your exercises and/or your system of training. The Rotational and Progressive system takes all this into account.

Reduce your reps and/or sets – Try doing just one work set instead of two and working within a lower rep range. Again, this is taken into consideration in the training steps 1 to 4.

Get an extra hour's sleep and reduce or drop your aerobic sessions – I know this sounds a bit vague, but you must understand that, although there are basic laws that apply to exercise progression, you are an individual. You have your own unique genetic make-up and your own unique lifestyle and commitments. Therefore, getting the right combination of exercise, rest and nutrition will be slightly different for you to the next person. Not only that, but you will also have different needs at different times of your life. For example, if you've just welcomed a baby into your family, your quality of sleep will be affected and you will have to modify your training and rest accordingly.

Listen to your body – Do you have a genuine need for rest or are you being idle? Having learned about overtraining, please do not use it as an excuse to take it easy. If you want to progress, you will have to work hard – very hard. I guess what I am really saying is work hard, but also work 'smart'. Hard work must be followed by complete recovery. Training is not an exact science and the pressures of life change from week to week. Be aware of this and manage your training and rest accordingly.

The information in this section should be read and re-read. A good understanding of this information is a major factor in productive long-term training. Small steady increments are the key to long-term success and your training enjoyment.

stretching – to do or not to do

Stretching is definitely a useful exercise when done properly and in the appropriate situations.

when should you stretch?

1. At the end of your session when the muscles are warm

2. As part of a rehabilitation programme after injury

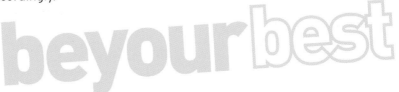

how should you stretch?

All stretches should be held for 20 to 30 seconds for best effect.

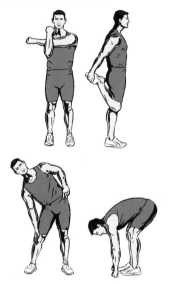

DOMS, or delayed onset of muscle soreness

This is a stiffness in the muscles that is sometimes experienced one or two days after a heavy training session. It happens to people who are exercising for the first time, or coming back to exercising after a long lay-off. It can also happen to well-trained people who change their exercise plan or do any other strenuous activity they are not used to. Some people say that it can be avoided by cooling down properly and stretching, but, although these are important parts of training, I do not believe they will always prevent DOMS occurring.

Nobody has completely explained why it happens, but, in my experience, it is short-lived and is just a part of the adaptation process to any new activity.

what to do when illness strikes

Many illnesses, especially colds and flulike illnesses, are the result of doing too much. You must learn to pace yourself. If you do become ill you should stop training immediately and get some rest. Training when ill is not advisable for the following reasons:

● Your training will be nonproductive and below par.

● You will either prolong or worsen your illness.

● You are more likely to injure yourself, which may prolong your time out of the gym long after your illness has cleared up.

Do not go back into the gym until you are 100 per cent well. Doing so may cause a relapse and put you right back to square one.

If you start getting regular bouts of minor illnesses like sore throats, cold sores or ulcers in the mouth, then I suggest you look at your training-to-rest ratio and your lifestyle in general. My guess is that you are overdoing it, and need more recovery time.

When you are better, go back to training steadily but look at what modifications need to be made (this is where your training diary will be invaluable).

The Rotational and Progressive system of training combines diet, exercise, rest and recovery and does the thinking for you.

9

the rotational and progressive system

> **'If the progression is slow enough and the body is given enough time for recovery along with adequate nutrition, adaptation will occur'**

introduction

According to Greek mythology, Milo of Croton was the first person to apply the theory of progressive overload training (550BC). He was an Olympic wrestler, who in his teens decided to become the strongest man in the world. He trained by lifting and carrying a baby bull every day; as the calf grew and became heavier, Milo became stronger. Finally, when the calf had developed into a full-grown bull, Milo, thanks to a long-term progression, was able to lift the huge beast. Consequently he became the strongest man on earth.

I do not know if this story is true, but I do know that the theory is sound.

Let's now get into the four-step plan of action and look at what you need to be doing in terms of training. We have already discussed CV and strength training and the merits of each. If you want low body fat, good shape, strength and high levels in heart and lung fitness, you will need to include both types of training. Add recovery and good nutrition to the mix and you have a system that will allow you to be your best.

the key to a successful training system

While I have prepared specific programmes and diet plans to suit each phase of the Rotational and Progressive method, it's important to understand what you're doing and why.

Everyone should start off easy (step 1) and slowly build momentum. If you are new to training you MUST spend the first phase learning correct exercise technique, building a base level of fitness and integrating smart eating into your life. Think of it in the same way you would think about building the foundations for a house. A good foundation is your first key to long-term success.

For those of you that already train regularly, this will be an opportunity to try a new system that will enable you to break plateaus and work towards your best condition ever.

Have a system and work it. The best system is one that gives you consistent gains. Not fast gains – consistent gains. If you try to add 2.5kg (5½lb) to the bar every week you will initially make some progress, especially if you are new to training. However, if you persist with this strategy your gains will soon dry up and you will hit a sticking point. Think about it: if you were training twice a week and increasing the bar by 2.5kg (5½lb) every session that would be 5kg (11lb) every week or 260kg (572lb) a year! Not possible! Therefore, we need to know what is achievable and what is the best possible strategy for long-term gains.

Get into the habit of recording everything you do in training. It is the key to keeping motivated and the key to understanding what works for you. I have training diaries going back as early as 1980, and have frequently referred to them. You simply cannot remember everything you do. It is much easier to analyse your training when you have a written record.

training diary

Your training diary is the place where you plan your strategy, record your results and make alterations if they are needed. It is your personal record and one of your most

powerful tools for continued progress and motivation.

Every year I go on a walking trip up in the Lake District with a group of friends. The trip involves arriving at a rented house on a specific day at a specific time. It involves having enough food for the five days, the right maps and all essential equipment. For the trip to be a success we plan out everything right down to the last detail. We work out all of the things that could go wrong and know exactly what to do in any adverse situation.

In other words, we have a basic blueprint that we follow and a list of coping strategies if things do not quite go to plan. Without these two things our walk would be random and very dangerous.

Your training diary is the place where you will plan your ongoing strategy. It will include your blueprint for success. It will be the place where you record your efforts and analyse your results. If progress slows it will show you how to change your plans: eat less/more, rest more/less, change your exercises, or a combination of these things. It will then allow you to analyse and change as often as you need, providing you keep it up to date.

You are a unique individual and the knowledge in this book gives you training, diet and recovery principles. The information in your training diary will make those principles specific to you. Your diary will show you what exercises, what rep ranges, what training cycles and what diets you personally respond to best.

My training diaries, over the years, have proved a valuable tool in my continued progress. Winning five Commonwealth Games over a twenty-year period did not happen by accident. I planned every session and learned over the years what worked and what did not. Without a training diary I would not have had the knowledge I needed to get the best out of myself. Do not make the mistake of thinking you will be able to remember, because, believe me, you will not.

Combine the knowledge in this book and the plans I'm giving you with the knowledge in your diary and you will enjoy long and continued progress that will enable you to be your best. That's guaranteed.

training methods

Circuit training

Moving without rest from one exercise to another until you have completed all exercises.

super set training

Alternating two exercises that work opposing muscle groups with no rest between sets. For example, seated press alternated with lat pull downs.

straight set training

Doing all of the sets of one exercise with 30 to 90 seconds' rest between sets and then moving to the next exercise.

In steps 1 to 3, you will be training twice per week. These sessions should be evenly spaced, for example, Monday and Thursday, or Tuesday and Friday, etc.

Note: If you do not have access to all the machines you can substitute with an exercise that works the same muscle groups (see Chapter 7).

step 1
duration – 8 weeks

Step 1 is designed to achieve the following:

● Learn correct exercise form

● Develop a base level of fitness (Strength and CV)

● Understand and incorporate the basics of smart eating

beyourbest

This is achieved by:

- **Circuit training using weights**

- **Progressive CV using bike and rower**

method

If you are new to exercise this step is about learning correct exercise technique and building a base level of fitness. This phase lasts for eight weeks and should be split into four two-week cycles.

Remember, circuit training involves moving from one exercise to the next without any rest.

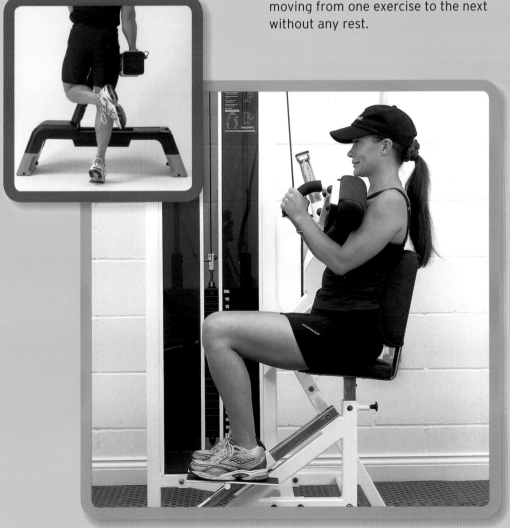

circuit 1

Weeks 1 to 2 are spent learning the exercises in circuit 1.

You will complete one circuit of all exercises in this cycle during weeks 1 and 2. Your session will start with 10 minutes on the bike at 65 per cent of your maximum heart rate and end with some stretching.

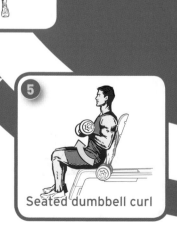

8

Calf raise

7

Leg press

6

Lateral raises

5

Seated dumbbell curl

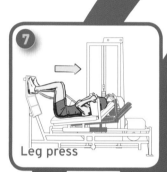

aerobic training		
Exercise	Time	Intensity*
Bike	10 minutes	65%

strength training		
Training Method	Repetition Range	Circuits
Circuit	10	1

*see page 65

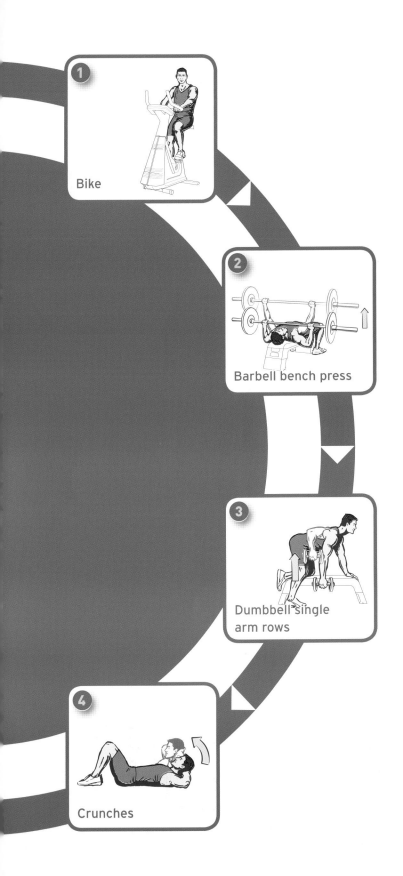

1 Bike

2 Barbell bench press

3 Dumbbell single arm rows

4 Crunches

circuit training
weeks 1-2

circuit 2

Weeks 3 to 4 are spent learning the exercises in circuit 2.

You should complete two circuits of all exercises in this cycle. Increase the aerobic training to 15 minutes and end with some stretching.

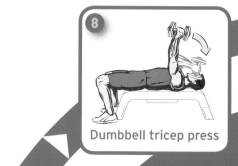

8 Dumbbell tricep press

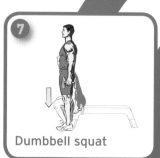

7 Dumbbell squat

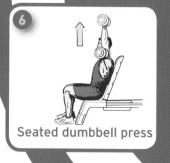

6 Seated dumbbell press

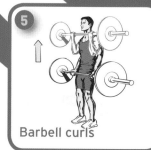

5 Barbell curls

aerobic training		
Exercise	Time	Intensity*
Bike	15 minutes	65-75%

strength training		
Training Method	Repetition Range	Circuits
Circuit	10	2

*see page 65

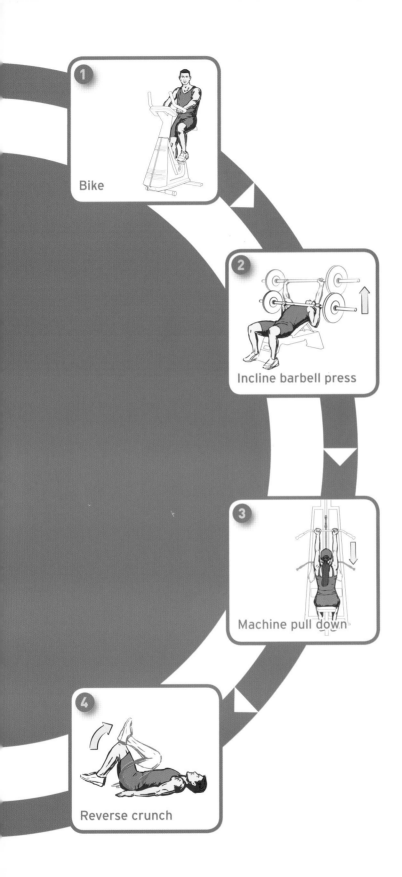

circuit training
weeks 3–4

1 Bike

2 Incline barbell press

3 Machine pull down

4 Reverse crunch

circuit 3

Weeks 5 to 6 are spent learning the exercises in circuit 3. Increase the aerobic training to 20 minutes and end with some stretching.

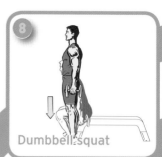

Dumbbell squat

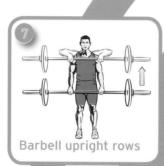

Barbell upright rows

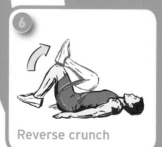

Reverse crunch

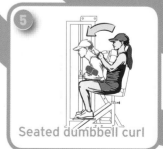

Seated dumbbell curl

Aerobic Training		
Exercise	Time	Intensity*
Bike	15 minutes	65–75%

Strength Training		
Training Method	Repetition Range	Circuits
Circuit	10	2

*see page 65

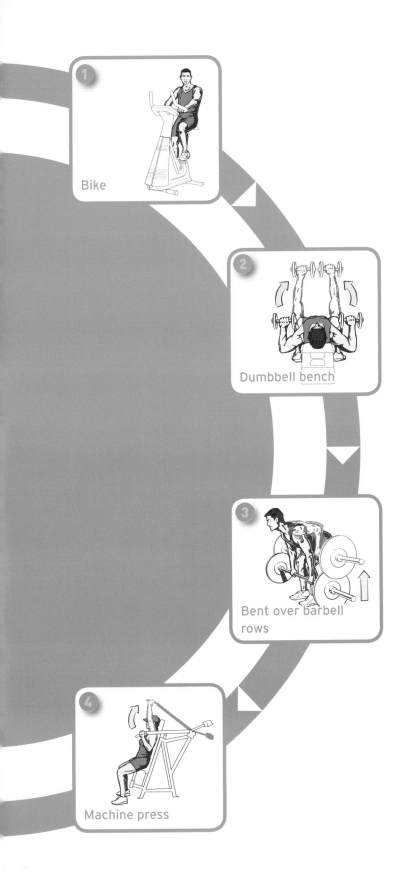

circuit training
weeks 5–6

1 Bike

2 Dumbbell bench

3 Bent over barbell rows

4 Machine press

circuit 4

Weeks 7-8 are spent learning the exercises in circuit 4.

Keep the aerobic training at 20 minutes but increase the intensity. In other words, work at the higher end of your heart-rate range.

A note on aerobics – as you become fitter you will have to increase the intensity to reach the required heart rate. There are two beneficial points to this:

1. Your cardiovascular system is becoming more efficient.

2. You are able to burn more calories in the same time, which means that your workouts will become more productive. This principle also applies to the weight training.

By now you will have a good understanding of the exercises and have developed a base level of fitness that you can build on. You will also have adopted healthier eating habits and, if you've stuck to my menu examples, you will already be noticing the benefits.

aerobic training		
Exercise	Time	Intensity*
Bike	20 minutes	75-85%

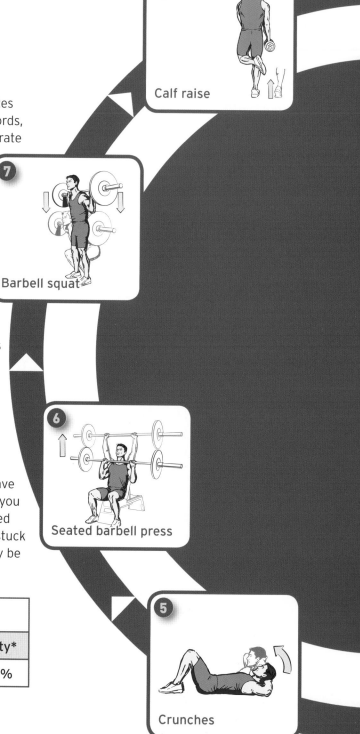

8 Calf raise

7 Barbell squat

6 Seated barbell press

5 Crunches

*see page 65

circuit training weeks 7-8

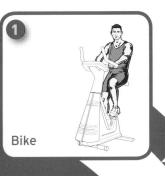

1 Bike

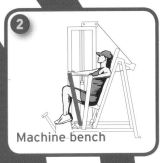

2 Machine bench

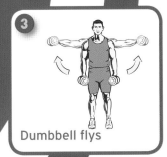

3 Dumbbell flys

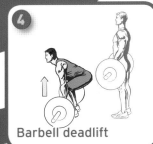

4 Barbell deadlift

strength training		
Training Method	Repetition Range	Circuits
Circuit	10	2

step 2
duration – 8 weeks

Step 2 is designed to achieve the following:

● Build on the base level

● Increase physical strength

● Improve CV fitness

This is achieved by:

● Lower repetitions

● Progressive weights

● Interval rows

Straight set training is when you complete the required repetitions of a particular exercise, and then rest for 60 to 90 seconds before completing your next set. When you have completed the required sets, move on to the next exercise.

aerobic training		
Exercise	Time	Intensity*
Interval rows	2 minutes on, 1 minute off, x 4	80-90%

strength training		
Training Method	Repetition Range	Work Sets
Straight sets	8-12	2

method

Start with your interval rows.

Take a five-minute rest, then begin your strength training. Select a weight that is about 50 per cent of your maximum for 12 repetitions. Example – if you can do 100kg (220lb) for 12 reps then you would start with 50kg (110lb) and do 12 repetitions; this is your first warm-up set. Now increase to 80 per cent – 80kg (176lb) in our example – and do 6 repetitions. Your warm-up is now complete and you are ready to begin.

Please note that the warm-up sets do not count as work sets.

Now choose a weight that you can do 8 to 12 reps on. If you cannot do 8 reps the weight is too heavy and if you can do more than 12 it is too light. Start with a weight that is hard in the lower rep range. As you get stronger you will find you are able to increase the repetitions to the higher rep range. When this happens you must increase the weight to bring yourself back into the lower rep range. In the beginning this will happen often. Strength gains of 50 to 100 per cent in the first year of training are normal. There is a certain amount of trial and error in the initial weight selection. This is normal and you will soon find your mark.

You need to maintain the number of reps throughout step 2 – therefore if you find that you are able to repeat more than 12 reps, you should up the weight.

*see page 65

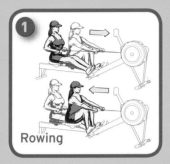

1 Rowing

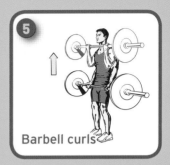

5 Barbell curls

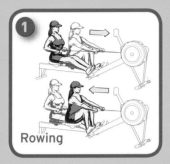

2 Barbell bench press

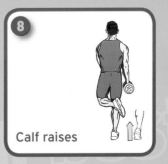

6 Crunches

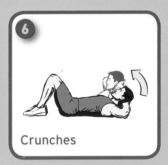

3 Barbell bent over rows

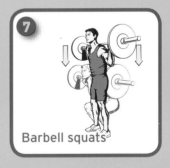

7 Barbell squats

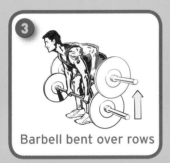

4 Barbell seated press

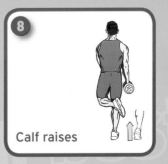

8 Calf raises

step 3
duration – 8 weeks

Step 3 is designed to achieve the following:

● Reduce body fat further

● Increase general fitness (strength and CV)

● Be able to do more work in less time

This is achieved by:

● Medium reps

● Super sets

● Higher-intensity aerobics

Super set training is when you group two exercises together that work opposing muscle groups and alternate them, without rest, until you have completed the required number of sets. Then move on to the next two grouped exercises.

aerobic training		
Exercise	Time	Intensity*
Rower/bike	20 Mins	75-85%

strength training		
Training Method	Repetition Range	Work Sets
Super sets	10-15	2

*see page 65

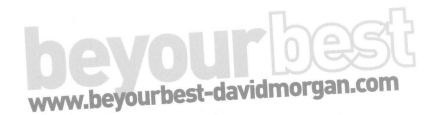

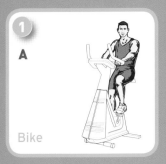

1

A

Bike

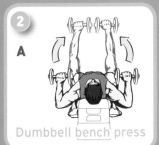

2

A

Dumbbell bench press

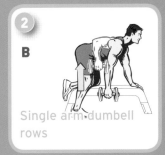

2

B

Single arm dumbell rows

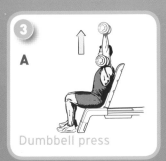

3

A

Dumbbell press

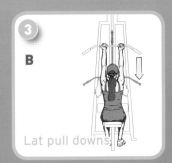

3

B

Lat pull downs

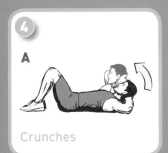

4

A

Crunches

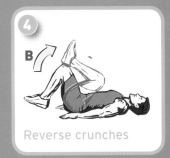

4

B

Reverse crunches

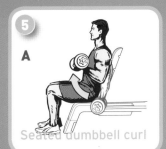

5

A

Seated dumbbell curl

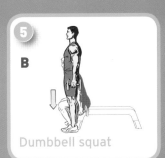

5

B

Dumbbell squat

The duration of each of the first three steps when you start is 8 weeks. That means it will take you 24 weeks to complete. By this time you should be in good shape and ready to move on to step 4.

step 4 – specialising

Because each person has different goals and needs it is at this point we can direct our training in a more specific way.

maintenance

Some of you will be happy with your condition now and just want to maintain it.

This can be done by simply going back through the three steps, this time spending six weeks on each step instead of eight.

At the end of this eighteen-week phase you should take a week off and then start again. For even more variety you can change the exercise you use in each cycle.

fat loss

I appreciate that you are all starting from different points and that some of you may still have body fat to lose. If this is the case you should follow the maintenance plan above, but with two changes:

1. Increase aerobic training to four times per week

2. Eat only fibrous carbohydrates with lunch and dinner

Note – once you have achieved your fat-loss goals, you can reduce the aerobic work to twice a week and go back to the normal smart-eating plan.

muscle gain

For those of you who are looking to gain muscle mass you should now make the following changes:

1. Drop the aerobic training completely

2. Increase your protein intake – you can do this by adding an extra protein shake before bed

3. Begin the following training programme outlined below

training day 1 – monday

exercise	reps	sets
Barbell squat	20	1
Barbell bench press	8-12	2
Bent over barbell rows	8-12	2
Weighted crunches	8-12	2

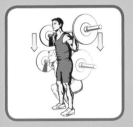
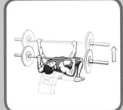
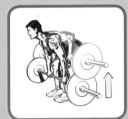
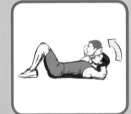

training day 2 – thursday

exercise	reps	sets
Barbell squat	20	1
Barbell dead lift	8-12	2
Seated barbell press	8-12	2
Standing barbell curl	8-12	2

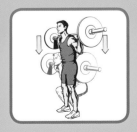
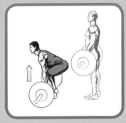
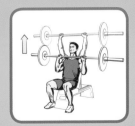
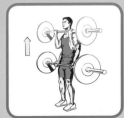

This is an abbreviated training routine, designed to increase size and strength. It is based around 20 rep squats - made popular by Randall Strossen's bestselling book *Super Squats*.

This training looks easy but, if it is done correctly, it is very demanding. The emphasis is on increasing the weights whenever you can, getting plenty of recovery and eating lots of the right types of food.

If after a month you are not making gains on this programme (by gains, I mean that the weights you are lifting are increasing), it may be you are not recovering properly. There are three possible reasons for this:

1. You are not resting enough in between sessions

2. You are not eating enough

3. A combination of both

First, make sure you are getting adequate rest between sessions. Make your initial training days Monday and Thursday. If your improvement slows down, try adding an extra rest day. Training would now be: session 1 Monday, session 2 Friday, session 1 Tuesday, session 2 Saturday, and so on.

Second, try adding an extra portion of carbohydrate in your first two meals and an extra portion of protein in your last meal of the day - this is in addition to the extra protein shake you have added already.

After six weeks on this routine, you should change over to the following routine to avoid getting stale.

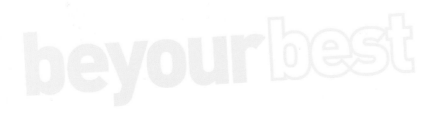

training day 1

exercise	reps	sets
Leg press	20	1
Incline barbell bench press	8-12	2
Barbell upright rows	8-12	2
Machine crunches	8-12	2

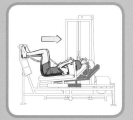
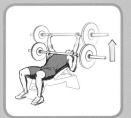
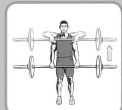
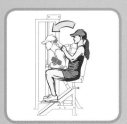

training day 2

exercise	reps	sets
Barbell squat	20	1
Barbell dead lift	8-12	2
Barbell upright rows	8-12	2
Machine crunches	8-12	2

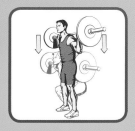
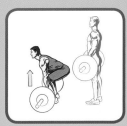
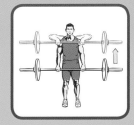
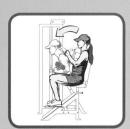

Continue alternating these routines and increasing the weights within the required rep range until you reach your strength and muscle gain goals. Once you have done this you can revert back to the Rotational and Progressive programme.

ectomorphs

There are some people out there who fall into a special body-type category. This category is called ectomorphic (see page 15). Ectomorphs will only gain muscle mass on a much-abbreviated training routine.

ectomorph training day 1

exercise	reps	sets
Barbell squat	20	1
Barbell bench press	8-12	2

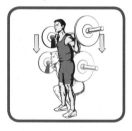
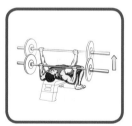

ectomorph training day 2

exercise	reps	sets
Deadlift	8-12	2
Barbell seated press	8-12	2
Barbell bent over rows	8-12	2

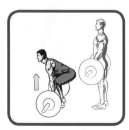
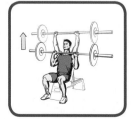
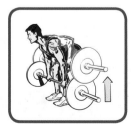

10

myths and

excuses

> Think back to all the skills and abilities you have developed so far in your life – learning to ride a bike, being taught how to swim or drive a car, learning a new language. Remember how difficult they all seemed at first and how easy they became once you had mastered the basics – almost second nature.

beyourbest

Well, developing a training programme is a new skill. At first it may seem hard, too difficult, an effort, and the end result may seem far away.

But don't be put off. You'll be amazed at the difference you can make. And it's not just a physical difference that you (and everyone else) will notice. You will find your mental attitude will also develop. You will become sharper, your concentration will improve, your confidence levels will soar and you will feel mentally fitter.

Of course there will be times when you would rather not work through your programme. We all have these moments and during those times it can be difficult to find the motivation. However, don't forget that every time you exercise you are taking one step closer to achieving your goal. And you will soon begin to notice the difference. The key to maintaining your momentum is to celebrate your short-term achievements.

Being in control and making the effort on those days when you do not feel like it will make the difference between achieving your goal or not. The sense of achievement you will experience by completing your programme for that day will far outweigh any feelings of relief you may feel by avoiding it - and you won't get the guilt, either.

So if you really can't get up half an hour earlier, or resist the takeaway three times a week, or talk yourself out of half your training sessions, your goal to be your best will be as far away as ever.

Here are some common myths and excuses.

'I have no time'

This is a good one. It is so easy to convince ourselves that our lives are too full to take on more. No time is a popular excuse and in today's busy world many people feel justified in using it.

Getting and staying in shape only requires two to three hours per week if you know what you are doing. Some of my most motivated clients are amongst the most 'time poor' – company directors and mums with young families.

I start work as early as 5 a.m. to cater for these motivated and successful people and they always turn up. They understand how important their health and fitness is, so they find the time.

'I'm too old to start'

It's never too late to benefit from properly structured exercise and a change in your diet. People's ability to make tremendous gains, even into their eighties, not only amazes me, but also gives me a great feeling of optimism for the future. All of my clients are over thirty – my eldest is eighty. Why do they train and eat well? Because it makes them feel good, look good and improves their quality of life.

'weight training will make me big and slow'

Weights are a tool that can be used to develop you in many different ways. Athletes use them to develop speed. Take a look at the 100m Olympic final. Those athletes did not get like that by just running. They understand that muscle means strength and that more strength means more speed. Many athletes spend just as much time in the weights room as on the track.

Weights can make you big if that's what you want. For the ladies reading this book, please note that weight training will not make you big, as you simply do not have enough of the male hormone testosterone.

By incorporating weight training into your programme, you will benefit from:

1. Increased strength

2. Improved shape and muscle tone

3. Maintained muscles – this is very important because, as you've already read, loss of muscle causes the metabolism to slow down, which in turn makes you more prone to fat gain.

Bingo wings (the affectionate name for the accumulation of fat that women often develop on the back of the upper arms as they get older) can be avoided by maintaining the muscle in this area. Weight training is also good for maintaining bone strength, which is particularly important for women going through the menopause.

'If I stop training my muscles will turn to fat'

Muscle does not turn to fat, it burns fat. Muscle and fat are two different compounds, which makes it impossible for one to change into the other. It is possible to gain muscle and lose body fat, and it is also possible to lose muscle and simultaneously gain fat if you stop training and start eating more calories than you need – but, I repeat, muscle does not turn to fat. It is a myth.

'aerobics is best for burning fat'

Many people think aerobic training is best for fat loss because fat is the main fuel used when working aerobically.

This is true, but you must ask yourself this question: 'How much time can I or do I want to spend doing aerobic training?'

My guess is not much more than 20 minutes 2 to 4 times per week. This will burn on average 250 calories per session. One pound of fat is equivalent to 3,500 calories, or 14 hours of aerobic work!

The truth is that hours of aerobic work coupled with the crazy diets found in magazines will turn you into a fat-making machine. That's a pretty hard statement to swallow, but it's true. Weight training burns little fat while you are training, but it does build muscle, which in turn burns fat 24 hours a day, and means you'll lose more fat when you're training and when you're not.

'I am on a diet and don't need to train'

Diets do not last forever. A diet is a temporary restriction of food that will cause muscle as well as fat loss, especially if you are not exercising. Eventually you will go off the diet and get back into your old habits. Because of the loss of muscle it will now take less food to make you fat. People that continually go on and off extreme diets find it more difficult to lose the weight each time, because of the muscle loss. This yo-yo dieting is very demoralising and can only end in failure, followed by more failure. You are literally training your body to get fat on less food.

The only way to break the cycle is to use weights to get back the lost muscle, which will put your metabolism back where it should be, and start eating smart.

Remember:

● Diets make you fat long term

● Training keeps you strong and young

'I'm in good shape, so I don't need to train any more'

Weight training makes you strong and can build and maintain muscle. As we get older we lose muscle and strength, which in turn makes us susceptible to fat gain. Regular weight-training sessions can stop and even reverse this part of the ageing process.

If you stop training, your body will notice and start to deteriorate. Use it or lose it.

'eating smart is expensive and time-consuming'

If you eat in the way I have suggested in Chapter 4, you will also be eating cheaper and spend less time preparing your food. Once you have changed your eating habits – and it doesn't take long to get into healthy eating – I can guarantee you will also look forward to your meals more.

If you decide you want to lose fat, gain strength and improve your quality of life – and you are obviously seriously considering it as you've bought this book – then get on and do it. Stop making excuses!

11

summary

> If you've read all the chapters, you are now in a position to fully understand the benefits of eating healthily and training regularly.

Whatever your objectives, this book will help you achieve them if you really want to.

If you are just used to feeling crap all the time you will be amazed how good you can feel.

If you have reached a plateau with your training it is possible to start to improve again, just by making small adjustments to your training and eating.

If you have been adopting fad diet after fad diet you will now know that it doesn't work long term. Well done for buying this book - follow the plan and notice the improvements - long term.

In reality, the only way to lose fat, feel better and improve your quality of life is to make small changes to your lifestyle. There is no magic formula - but you can take control and make it happen.

The more fat you want to lose or the more muscle you have to build, the longer it will take you to reach your goal, but your gains may be visible sooner.

Personally, I want to enjoy my life to the full, and live better, for longer.

I really believe that you can be your best - wherever you're at right now. Follow the Progressive and Rotational system, record your training and eating, regularly re-evaluate what you're doing, make the necessary tweaks to the programme, and enjoy the results.

about david

David Morgan is a five-times Commonwealth weightlifting champion. From the age of thirteen, David has competed, and consistently won, at a world level.

He has the distinction of being the only athlete from any sport, and any of the 71 competing nations, to win this many Commonwealth Games in history. He has also competed in three Olympic Games and is the current World Masters Champion and holds five world records.

Trained in Sports Psychology, Physiology, Biomechanics and Nutrition, David also now works as a personal trainer and a sports commentator for the satellite channel Eurosport and has commentated on the World Championships, European Championships and the Olympic Games.

David owns a 2,000-square-feet personal-training facility in Cambridge, and remains very close to the world of weightlifting, coaching the British Masters team - which boasts five gold medallists and four world record holders.

David is, however, an ordinary bloke who has combined determination, motivation, his own money and a lot of hard work to achieve his objectives.

He has been at the top of his sport for over 25 years, and now, at the age of 42, continues to maintain and enjoy his training and healthy-eating regime to keep him at the peak of physical health.

David is heavily involved in charity work, helping to raise over £1m during the last five years for several charities, and in 2005 beat Brian Jacks twenty-year-old *Superstars* dips record, by achieving an incredible 102 dips in 54 seconds, while raising money for Comic Relief.

successes

Date	Competition	Place	Bodyweight	Snatch	Clean & Jerk	Age
1979	British Schoolboy	1st	48kg	70kg	90kg	14
1980	Junior World Championships	10th	56kg	87.5kg	112.5kg	15
1981	Junior World Championships	10th	60kg	105kg	132.5kg	16
1982	Junior World Championships	3rd	67.5kg	135kg	160kg	17
1982	Commonwealth Games	Gold	67.5kg	132.5kg	162.5kg	18 and a day
1984	Olympic Games	4th	75kg	145kg	185kg	19
1984	Junior World Championships	2nd	75kg	150kg	180kg	19
1986	Commonwealth Games	Gold	82.5kg	160kg	190kg	21
1986	European Championships	4th	75kg	155kg	190kg	21
1987	British Championships	1st	82.5kg	160kg	205kg	22
1987	European Championships	3rd	82.5kg	165kg	200kg	22
1988	Olympic Games	4th	82.5kg	165kg	200kg	23
1990	Commonwealth Games	Gold	82.5kg	155kg	192.5kg	25
1994	Commonwealth Games	Gold	76kg	147.5kg	180kg	29

2000	World Masters	1st	77kg	137.5kg	150kg	35
2001	European Masters	1st	77kg	140kg	160kg	36
2002	Commonwealth Games	Gold	77kg	145kg	160kg	37
2005	British Masters	1st	85kg	135kg	160kg	40
2005	World Masters	1st	85kg	140kg (world record)	162kg (world record)	40
2006	World Masters Championships	1st	77kg	126kg (world record)	145kg	41

best ever training lifts

Bodyweight 80kg

Snatch   170kg (374lb)

Clean and Jerk   207.5kg (456½lb)

Jerk from Racks   220kg (484lb)

Front Squat   230kg (506lb)

Back Squat   275kg (605lb)

Power Snatch   150kg (330lb)

Power Clean   170kg (374lb)

Power Clean   140kg (308lb)

Back Squat   180kg (396lb) x 20

Dead Lift   230kg (506lb) x 10

Bench Press   140kg (308lb) x 10

'Concept 2' 2000m rowing   6 minutes 35 seconds

Parallel bar dips   102 in one minute to beat the *Superstars* record set by Brian Jacks (Comic Relief BBC coverage 2005)

Weighted parallel bar dips   90kg (198lb) 10 reps

now (age 42)

David now takes a more all-round approach to his training.

Snatch   140kg (308lb)
(Masters world record)

Clean and Jerk   162kg   (356½lb)
(Masters world record)